Praise For Dr. Shekhar K. Challa and "Probiotics For Dummies"

"With *Probiotics For Dummies,* Dr. Shekhar Challa once again simplifies a complicated subject in a way that will help readers improve their health. This book is an excellent resource identifying current research in the probiotics field, and is easily understood and informative. It's a clear guide showing readers how and why it's important to incorporate probiotics in their diets."

> — Dr. Michael Sorrell
> Robert L. Grissom Professor of Medicine
> Section of Gastroenterology and Hepatology
> Co-director of Solid Organ Transplant Service
> University of Nebraska College of Medicine

"Don't let the humorous title *Probiotics For Dummies* mislead you. Dr Challa's very comprehensive primer will help you quickly grasp the vital importance of probiotics from both supplements and food. With easy-to-understand facts and the most recent medical research, you'll see why probiotics and prebiotics are the foundation for a long, healthy life."

> — Donna Gates
> Nutritional Consultant
> Author of *The Body Ecology Diet*

"Dr. Shekhar Challa's book, *Probiotics For Dummies*, provides an easy-to-understand, practical framework for learning about probiotics. Focusing on overall wellness, he demystifies the digestive realm of microflora, micronutrients, supplements, and medications, giving readers a 'go to' resource to make informed health decisions."

> — Mary Schluckebier, B.S., M.A.
> Executive Director
> Celiac Sprue Association

"Outstanding! Having read numerous books on probiotics in preparation for my new film on these 'good bugs,' I was extremely impressed with all the great and useful information provided in Dr. Challa's new book. His experience as a board-certified gastroenterologist clearly makes a huge difference in explaining to the reader how important probiotics are, not only for gastrointestinal health but for overall excellent health and wellbeing. I would highly recommend *Probiotics For Dummies* for anyone wishing to learn about these beneficial bacteria!"

> — David Knight
> Executive Producer,
> *Microwarriors: The Power of Probiotics*

"I can't think of a better gastroenterologist than Dr. Challa to navigate the tour through the new and powerful world of probiotics — from GI conditions and women's health issues to allergies and immunity. Certain probiotic strains can make the difference between health and illness, and *Probiotics For Dummies* covers it all in a user-friendly way.

> — Elaine Magee, M.P.H., R.D.
> Author of 25 books on nutrition, including *Tell Me What To Eat If I Have Acid Reflux* and *Tell Me What To Eat If I Have Irritable Bowel Syndrome*

Probiotics

FOR

DUMMIES®

Probiotics
FOR
DUMMIES®

by Dr. Shekhar K. Challa, M.D.
Board-Certified Gastroenterologist

Foreword by
Eamonn M. M. Quigley, M.D.,
F.R.C.P., F.A.C.P., F.A.C.G.,
F.R.C.P.I.
Professor of Medicine and
Human Physiology

WILEY

John Wiley & Sons, Inc.

Probiotics For Dummies®

Published by
John Wiley & Sons, Inc.
111 River St.
Hoboken, NJ 07030-5774
www.wiley.com

For general information on our other products and services, please contact our Customer Care Department within the U.S. at 877-762-2974, outside the U.S. at 317-572-3993, or fax 317-572-4002.

For technical support, please visit www.wiley.com/techsupport.

Wiley publishes in a variety of print and electronic formats and by print-on-demand. Some material included with standard print versions of this book may not be included in e-books or in print-on-demand. If this book refers to media such as a CD or DVD that is not included in the version you purchased, you may download this material at http://booksupport.wiley.com. For more information about Wiley products, visit www.wiley.com.

Library of Congress Control Number: 2012935730

ISBN: 978-1-118-16973-5

ISBN 978-1-118-22656-8 (ePDF); ISBN 978-1-118-23981-0 (ePub); ISBN 978-1-118-25488-2 (eMobi)

Manufactured in the United States of America

10 9 8 7 6 5 4 3 2 1

WILEY

About the Author

Dr. Shekhar Challa, M.D., is a board-certified gastroenterologist who has been at the forefront of gastroenterology and hepatology for 24 years. In private practice in Topeka, Kansas, since 1987, Dr. Challa is president of Kansas Medical Clinic and CEO of Osteoporosis Services, the largest mobile bone density testing company in the Midwest.

Dr. Challa also is the author of *Winning the Hepatitis C Battle*, which was a finalist for the Independent Book Publishers Association's Benjamin Franklin Awards, and *Spurn the Burn: Treat the Heat (Everything You Need to Know about Acid Reflux Disease)*. As a passionate advocate of education as a way to help people achieve the best quality of life, Dr. Challa has been interviewed extensively by national media, including *Seventeen* magazine, *Girl's Life*, and numerous radio and TV shows.

He has been a featured speaker for several pharmaceutical companies and has served on national and international boards, including those for West Central Osteoporosis-Proctor and Gamble, US Bank, AmSurg, and My Medical Records.com. He has been the principal investigator for several clinical trials for various pharmaceutical companies.

Dedication

To my dad, Somrajram Challa, who is going through a tough time right now with medical problems: It is from you that I learned the work ethic and dedication I bring to my career. Thank you for your loving guidance.

To my mother, Anantha Lakshmi: Thank you for the ability to cut to the heart of the matter that you bring to my life. I have never met anyone with more common sense than you have.

To Jaya, my patient wife, who supported me as I spent time writing this book, which was time I "took away" from you. To Akhila and Shruti, my beautiful daughters who mean the world to me.

Acknowledgments

Thank you to Morgan, Lily, and Akhila for countless meetings, emails, and hours of hard work and research putting this book together.

To Dr. Jessica Brown, a future gastroenterologist, for your research contributions. Wishing you good luck in your career path.

To Mark Brudnak, Ph.D, for being a great technical editor . . . and for keeping me in line, and to the Wiley "For Dummies" team, including CC, Tracy, Kim, and Meg.

To my nephews, Dr. Karthik Challa, Dr. Abishek Challa, Dr. Nitin Chandra Pendyala, and med school students Rudra Pampati, Abhinay Challa, Vinayak Pampati, and Abhiram Challa.

To aspiring physicians, undergraduate student Ms. Stephanie Downes and high school students Sahil Rattan, Nitish S. Chimalakonda, and Aparna Dasaraju, for helping to research.

To Cori and Quintin for playing devil's advocate on this project. To Julie Drick for transcribing many, many tapes over the last 14 months.

To all my staff at Kansas Medical Clinic and the Endoscopy Center of Topeka for re-orienting me when I was going crazy juggling work and this project.

Publisher's Acknowledgments

We're proud of this book; please send us your comments at http://dummies.custhelp.com. For other comments, please contact our Customer Care Department within the U.S. at 877-762-2974, outside the U.S. at 317-572-3993, or fax 317-572-4002.

Some of the people who helped bring this book to market include the following:

Acquisitions, Editorial, and Vertical Websites

Editor: CC Powell

Acquisitions Editor: Tracy Boggier

Assistant Editor: David Lutton

Editorial Program Coordinator: Joe Niesen

Technical Editor: Mark Brudnak, Ph.D.

Nutrition Analyst: Patty Santelli

Senior Editorial Manager: Jennifer Ehrlich

Editorial Manager: Carmen Krikorian

Editorial Assistant: Alexa Koschier

Art Coordinator: Alicia B. South

Cover Photos: Front: © iStockphoto.com / Sebastian Kaulitzki Back: © iStockphoto.com / Carolyn Woodcock

Cartoons: Rich Tennant (www.the5thwave.com)

Composition Services

Project Coordinator: Nikki Gee

Layout and Graphics: Melanee Habig, Joyce Haughey, Corrie Niehaus

Proofreader: John Greenough

Indexer: Slivoskey Indexing Services

Illustrator: Kathryn Born

Publishing and Editorial for Consumer Dummies

Kathleen Nebenhaus, Vice President and Executive Publisher

Kristin Ferguson-Wagstaffe, Product Development Director

Ensley Eikenburg, Associate Publisher, Travel

Kelly Regan, Editorial Director, Travel

Publishing for Technology Dummies

Andy Cummings, Vice President and Publisher

Composition Services

Debbie Stailey, Director of Composition Services

Contents at a Glance

Contents

Foreword

A medical historian of the future looking back at medical progress may well highlight the discovery of antibiotics as the great medical breakthrough of the 20th century; when that same historian looks back at the 21st century he or she may well come to recognize it as the era when the bugs fought back! What I am referring to is the *microbiome revolution*: the very exciting and ever-increasing knowledge being accumulated on how certain bacteria are a normal and, indeed, essential component of the human body. Bacteria contribute to our growth, development, and health to such an extent that some have come to refer to the microbiome (the collection of bugs in our gut) as the "hidden" or "ignored" organ.

As medical science, aided by rapid advances in technology, comes to recognize the true size and diversity of this microbiome and appreciate how it participates actively in such essential bodily functions as immunity and metabolism, the possibility that approaches that change the microbiota may be useful in treating disease has emerged. Indeed, the concept of giving "good" bacteria to alleviate common complaints as well as prevent or treat illness is not a new one, but has been practiced by communities around the world for centuries.

A number of approaches can be taken to impacting the bacteria in the gut; the first, of course, is by using antibiotics. This occurs inadvertently every time we take an antibiotic by mouth to treat a chest or urinary infection, for example, when the very same antibiotic that zaps the bad bug also suppresses the good bacteria in the gut, albeit transiently. This is a blunderbuss strategy; much subtler is the approach that aims to selectively increase the numbers of certain good bacteria by either administering them directly (as a probiotic supplement) or attempting to promote their growth by giving specific foods (prebiotics) that achieve this.

While the science behind probiotics is now considerable, the consumer who goes into a store seeking help continues to face many challenges. When should I consider a probiotic? What one should I take? Does a given product contain what it claims? Does it really work? What is the best way to take it? When attempting to answer these questions, the consumer is confronted by much hype — unsupported claims presented as sound evidence. Until regulatory processes are put in place which assist the consumer and the health care professional in choosing the right probiotic for a given problem, confusion will be inevitable. This is where this book by Dr. Challa — an eminent clinician and expert in gastrointestinal disorders and the field of probiotics — steps in by providing an accessible, critical, yet practical guide to the perplexing topic of probiotics.

In this book he provides a very helpful background to probiotics in general and then takes the reader on a journey through the many areas in medicine and health where probiotics may have a place, concluding with helpful hints on the use or probiotics in daily life. His discussion of each area of potential use of a probiotic is set clearly in the context of a specific clinical problem, the rationale for the use of a probiotic is presented, and the merits and shortcomings of probiotic therapy are discussed. What emerges is a balanced and eminently readable book that should be of value to all those who wish to learn more about this exciting topic.

Dr. Eamonn M. M. Quigley,
Professor of Medicine and Human Physiology,
Alimentary Pharmabiotic Centre,
University College Cork, Ireland

Introduction

● ●

*M*ost people have experienced occasional digestive trouble — diarrhea, constipation, and so on. Between 15 million and 30 million Americans suffer from *irritable bowel syndrome* (see Chapter 2), and many millions more are affected by a range of other digestive disorders. For many years, such people either got by with no treatment at all or used prescription and over-the-counter medications that, too often, either didn't work or didn't work well enough.

Fortunately, researchers now understand much more about how your body's digestive system actually works. As it turns out, your intestines are populated by hundreds of different kinds of bacteria — some of which cause problems, but most of which are *good* bacteria, keeping the bad guys under control and performing vital functions for your immune system and overall health.

As this body of knowledge has grown, so have efforts to create products that help your body keep that critical balance of good bacteria alive and thriving. *Probiotics* are good bacteria, and they're showing up more and more frequently in foods and in dietary supplements.

About This Book

This book is intended to be a handy primer on how probiotics work, why they help keep you healthy, and how they can affect certain health problems. One chapter even covers the most recent findings on the role probiotics may play in preventing or treating diseases such as colon cancer and cardiovascular disease.

Although various societies throughout history have used probiotics in one form or another (more on this in Chapter 1), their use in the United States is relatively recent, and reliable, easy-to-understand information about probiotics can be hard to come by.

This book is designed to help fill the need for good information about probiotics and to answer basic questions about how they may benefit you.

In some cases, the research about probiotics is promising but incomplete. I explain the promise and the possibilities, but when those promises and possibilities aren't yet proven, I caution that more research is needed.

Conventions Used in This Book

For the sake of consistency and readability, I use the following conventions throughout the text:

- ✔ Technical terms appear in *italics*, with a plain-English definition or explanation nearby.
- ✔ Keywords in bulleted lists and the action part of numbered steps are in **bold.**

When this book was printed, some Web addresses may have been split into two lines of text. If that happened, rest assured that I haven't inserted any extra characters (such as hyphens) to indicate the break. So, when using one of these Web addresses, just type exactly what you see in this book as though the line break doesn't exist.

What You're Not to Read

Occasionally, you'll see sidebars — shaded boxes of text that go into detail on a particular topic. You don't have to read them if you're not interested; skipping them won't hamper your understanding the rest of the text.

You also can skip any information next to the Technical Stuff icon. I explain most technical information in simple language and reserve the Technical Stuff icon for details that are interesting but not crucial to understanding the topic.

Foolish Assumptions

In researching and writing this book, I've made some assumptions about you, the reader. I assume that you

- ✔ Have a health condition (or a loved one with a health condition) for which probiotics may provide effective treatment.

- ✔ Want to know how probiotics can help improve and maintain your overall health and wellbeing.

- ✔ Are interested in how gut health may affect other health issues and concerns.

- ✔ Would like to know how to select effective probiotic supplements and how to fill your plate with probiotic-rich foods.

- ✔ Want a convenient, comprehensive, and easy-to-understand resource that covers all this information without making you feel like a dummy.

How This Book Is Organized

The information in this book is split into broad subtopics so you can easily find the stuff you want. I divided the subject of probiotics into the following parts.

Part 1: Living in the Microbial World

This part focuses on the scientific foundations for probiotics' role in combating disease and promoting overall good health.

This part includes a chapter on your digestive system to help you understand both the friendly and unfriendly microbes in your body. I also provide a chapter that gives you an overview of probiotics and prebiotics.

Part II: Preserving and Improving Health with Probiotics

This part covers the nitty gritty of probiotics' role in health. Starting with digestive health, I follow up with the latest research on how probiotics may affect a plethora of other ailments and diseases, including allergies, urogenital infections, and women's and children's health.

I also cover the latest research on some really exciting possibilities for probiotics: fighting such common conditions as heart disease, certain forms of cancer, and even autoimmune diseases such as diabetes.

Part III: Adding Probiotics to Your Lifestyle

This part gives you information on probiotics-rich foods as well as a collection of recipes for making your own probiotic-rich meals, snacks, condiments, and desserts.

Part IV: The Part of Tens

The Part of Tens is a staple of every *For Dummies* book; the information here is presented in bite-sized nuggets for a quick and easy read.

Here, I present a quick look at Ten Ways Probiotics Promote Good Health, Ten Common Misconceptions About Probiotics, and Ten Famous Bacteria.

Icons Used in This Book

Occasionally throughout the text, you see little icons in the left-hand margin. Here's what these symbols mean:

This symbol alerts you to information that's important to keep in mind as you explore using probiotics.

The bull's-eye icon indicates helpful information, such as how to choose probiotics-rich foods or where to find probiotic supplements.

Okay, nothing is *really* going to explode if you don't heed the information next to this little bomb. But it does tell you that you should be aware of potential problems.

Technical Stuff is information that's interesting but not essential; you can safely skip over text marked with this icon without missing anything important.

Where to Go from Here

Like all *For Dummies* books, this one is organized so that you can find the information that matters to you and ignore the stuff you don't care about. You don't have to read the chapters in any particular order; each chapter contains the information you need for that chapter's topic, and I provide cross-references if you want to read more about a specific subject. You don't even have to read the entire book (but I'd be delighted if you do).

To learn more about how your digestive system works and the good bacteria that help it function properly, turn to Chapter 2. If you're ready to start making probiotic meals at home, check out the recipes in Chapter 12. If you want to know how probiotics may help your children stay healthier, flip to Chapter 8. And if you want to discover how probiotics may be involved in heart health, cancer prevention, and a host of other health issues, go to Chapter 9.

Part I

Living in the Microbial World

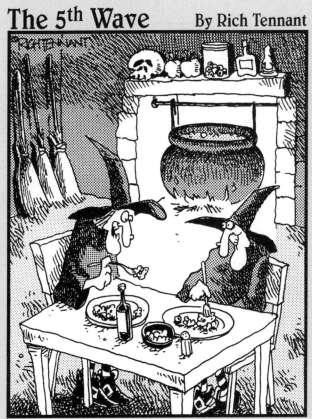

The 5th Wave   By Rich Tennant

"I substitute yogurt for eye of newt nowadays. It has half the calories and doesn't wriggle around the cauldron."

In this part . . .

1 explore the basics of how bacteria — good and bad — impact your body and its functions. From your immune system to your intestines, bacteria affect your health in numerous ways. Understanding the basics of that impact will help you understand how probiotics can help you not only achieve better health but also fight some diseases. Lastly, I help you understand what probiotics are and what you'll look for as you incorporate this important supplement into your diet.

Chapter 1

Getting a Handle on the True Nature of Bacteria

*T*he United States, the world leader in so many other areas of health and medical science, is considered an "emerging market" in the development and use of probiotics; such supplements are far more popular in Europe and Asia, and probiotic-rich foods (see Chapter 11) are staples in many cultures around the globe.

Interestingly, according to the National Health Interview Survey conducted by the National Institutes of Health's National Center for Complementary and Alternative Medicine (http://nccam.nih.gov), Americans use probiotics for their children, but not for themselves. Certainly, children can benefit from probiotics (see Chapter 8), but research indicates that probiotics are appropriate for grown-ups too. Even healthy adults can help maintain their good health by taking probiotics.

As in other countries, yogurt manufacturers in the United States have long touted the benefits of live cultures of bacteria in their products. More recently, companies like Dannon have begun aggressively marketing yogurt and its friendly bacteria as a way to regulate your digestive system — and they back up their claims by financing or conducting clinical studies.

The National Center for Complementary and Alternative Medicine also has made probiotic research a high priority for funding projects. The center supports research on using probiotics to alleviate or prevent various gastrointestinal disorders in infants and children; treating and preventing antibiotic-related diarrhea (see Chapter 4); and improving the efficacy of flu vaccines.

Government and privately funded research is turning up lots of evidence that probiotics can do more than regulate your digestive system. I provide information on various health applications for specific probiotic strains throughout this book. But researchers also are uncovering fascinating links between the bacteria in your digestive system and your brain's development, as well as mental health issues like anxiety and depression, which I discuss later in this chapter. First, though, the next section provides a brief overview of the theories and discoveries about bacteria's role in sickness and health.

Exploring the History of Bacteria Theories and Practices

Centuries before the invention of the microscope enabled researchers to observe living organisms that are invisible to the naked eye, some scientists theorized that tiny creatures spread disease among animals and humans. Ancient Hindu texts, for example, refer to living agents as causing disease. In 36 BC Marcus Terentius Varro warned against building homes and farms near swamps because such areas breed "certain minute creatures, which cannot be seen by the eyes, which enter the body through the mouth and nose and there cause serious diseases."

Even so, conventional wisdom discounted the idea that organisms like bacteria, or germs, caused illness. The prevalent theory was that disease generated spontaneously. Even Anton van Leeuwenhoek, considered the father of microbiology, didn't connect the organisms he saw under his microscope with disease. And the idea that human contact could transmit harmful microorganisms met with massive resistance among the medical and scientific communities.

In the following sections, I provide a brief overview of how the germ theory of disease developed and the history of using probiotics, or good bacteria, to promote good health.

Understanding germ theory

Although it forms the basis of medical treatment and hygiene practices today, *germ theory* — the idea that microorganisms are responsible for causing and spreading illness — was quite controversial for centuries. Before the invention of the microscope, most people (including most doctors and scientists) believed that disease either arose spontaneously or was spread through "bad air," or *miasma*.

Ignaz Semmelweis, a Hungarian obstetrician working at a Vienna hospital in 1847, noticed that when doctors and medical students attended births, new mothers were far more likely to die of *puerperal* fever, commonly known as childbed fever, than women who delivered their babies at home with the aid of a midwife. Semmelweis observed that doctors and medical students at the hospital often delivered babies right after performing autopsies, and he insisted that doctors wash their hands in a chlorinated solution before examining pregnant women. This elementary technique lowered the childbed fever death rate at the hospital from nearly 1 in 5 to about 1 in 50.

English physician John Snow added evidence supporting the germ theory when he traced the origins of a cholera outbreak in London in the 1850s. Snow noticed that the homes of people affected by the outbreak all got their water from the same pump, and he identified that water as the mechanism for spreading the disease.

In the 1860s, Louis Pasteur conducted experiments that proved that living organisms in freshly boiled broth came from outside the broth rather than spontaneously generating within it. A decade later, Joseph Lister (for whom the Listerine brand mouthwash is named) developed procedures for sterilizing surgical instruments and wounds in hospitals.

Although some physicians and scientists proposed some version of germ theory for centuries, the idea didn't gain wide acceptance until the late 19th century, when Robert Koch demonstrated that anthrax was caused by specific bacteria.

Since then, germ theory has led to development of antibiotics and hygiene standards, and it remains a foundational element of both modern medicine and microbiology.

Discovering probiotics' benefits

For more than a century, germ theory (see the preceding section) focused on the idea that bacteria caused disease. In fact, many common bacteria do cause illness in humans and animals, but many others are harmless, and still others are actually beneficial. Beneficial bacteria today are known as probiotics.

Years ago, scientists believed that human beings and the bacteria in their bodies had a *commensal* relationship — meaning that they exist together without harming each other. Advances in medicine helped to clarify that this relationship is *mutualistic;* that is, both your body and the bacteria in it benefit from each other.

The concept that some bacteria may promote health rather than harm it was born in the early 20th century when Russian scientist Eli Metchnikoff hypothesized that eating fermented milk products contributed to the long life span of Bulgarian peasants. He concluded that fermented milk helped to "seed" the intestine with friendly bacteria, which suppressed the growth of harmful bacteria.

Metchnikoff believed that lactic acid bacteria in milk contributed to the Bulgarian peasants' general health and long lives, and he was the first scientist to propose using these bacteria to prevent and treat certain illnesses. He also was the first to suggest that it's possible to modify the gut flora by replacing harmful bacteria with useful microorganisms, later winning a Nobel Prize for his work.

Every society has consumed some type of fermented food on a daily basis, and anthropologists theorize this practice dates from prehistoric times. As a food staple, cow's milk dates back at least 9,000 years, and some Central Asian people drank horse milk long before cows were domesticated. They stored milk in bladders made of animal intestines, and the microorganisms from the bladders fermented the milk into yogurt.

Marco Polo: Probiotics pioneer

Thirteenth-century explorer and tradesman Marco Polo, the first European to travel deep into the interior of China and Mongolia, mentioned *kefir*, a fermented milk drink, and its "magical properties," in his travel journals. Some historians think kefir may have contributed to the high survival rate among Marco Polo's sailors at a time when many seamen died of intestinal disorders.

Kefir is one of the oldest known fermented milk products, but it wasn't generally known outside the Caucasus region (at the border between Europe and Asia) until the 19th century. To learn more about kefir's interesting history, visit www.kefir.biz/history.htm.

Food historians note that yogurt was widely consumed in Central Asia, India, and the Middle East for thousands of years. Indian texts dating from around 6000 BC refer to the health benefits of milk and milk products, and modern Indian cuisine includes more than 700 kinds of yogurt and cheese products. As exploration opened up trade between Asia and Europe, yogurt and other fermented dairy products made their way into Europe and eventually to the New World. (See the nearby sidebar, "Marco Polo: Probiotics pioneer.")

Fermented milks are the best example of early probiotics. Milk turns sour in hot climates, so — especially in the days before refrigeration — many people deliberately fermented milk to make curd, or yogurt. Today, the same curd or yogurt is made in a controlled environment by adding live cultures such as *Lactobacillus acidophilus* or *Lactobacillus bulgaricus*.

Bacteria are categorized using Latin nomenclature that identifies genus and species. So *Lactobacillus* means a bacterium that produces lactic (or milk) acid, and *acidophilus* means the bacterium is a species that survives well in acid environments, such as your stomach.

Looking at Bacteria and the Brain

Recent research into how various bacteria interact with and affect systems outside the digestive tract has turned up intriguing connections between the brain and the gut.

For example, researchers at The Sage Colleges in Troy, New York, found that mice fed with a harmless strain of soil bacteria learned a new maze twice as fast as mice who weren't given the bacteria, and the bacteria-fed mice exhibited fewer signs of anxiety, such as grooming and searching (see "Controlling Mood and Anxiety" later in this chapter).

Meanwhile, a collaborative study between scientists at Karolinska Institutet in Sweden and the Genome Institute of Singapore indicates that gut bacteria may play a critical role in brain development, which influences adult behavior. The researchers compared behavior and *gene expression* — the way information in genes is translated and used to communicate with cells — between mice raised with normal gut bacteria and *germ-free* mice, which had no gut bacteria.

The germ-free mice were more active and exhibited more risky behaviors than the normal mice. When the germ-free mice were exposed to normal bacteria very early in life, their behavior as adults was closer to that of normal adult mice. But exposing the germ-free mice to these bacteria as adults had no effect on their behavior, indicating that bacteria play an important role in early brain development. In fact, the researchers identified significant differences in gene expression and signaling pathways between the two groups of mice; these differences involved learning, memory, and motor control.

The research team was careful to note that their findings apply only to mice, and it's too early to say whether gut bacteria play a similar role in human brain development. However, these findings open up intriguing possibilities for discovering just how big a role gut bacteria play in human physical development. (To understand why researchers use mice and other organisms to study human development and disease, see the nearby sidebar, "Of mice and humans.")

Of mice and humans

Researchers in many fields routinely experiment on mice before they develop clinical trials for humans because, biologically speaking, humans and mice have a lot in common. Cells in humans and mice (as well as fruit flies, yeasts, and many other animals and organisms) have a distinct nucleus encased in a membrane, and several genes are interchangeable between species.

Bacteria differ from humans, mice, and other organisms in that their cells don't have a compartmentalized nucleus. Instead, bacterial cells have a less-defined *nucleoid region* that contains their DNA.

Mouse models of human diseases give researchers important insights into how diseases develop and progress, as well as the molecular and genetic pathways involved. When scientists develop new drugs or therapies, they first test them on mice and other lab animals before moving onto clinical trials to assess their safety and effectiveness in humans.

Controlling Mood and Anxiety

Researchers also are investigating the relationship between bacteria in your digestive system and psychological issues, such as depression, stress, and anxiety. These connections also have implications for your immune system.

Scientists have learned a lot about how the different systems in your body communicate with each other, but they're far from fully understanding the complexities of that communication. The idea that gut bacteria play a role in systemic communications is relatively new, and most studies have so far been done only in mice or rats, not in humans. However, these studies open up fascinating possibilities for treating a host of physical and psychological issues.

In the following sections, you discover how stress can impact your immune system by changing the composition of your gut bacteria, as well as the potential links between probiotic bacteria and mood and anxiety.

Stressing out your immune system

Medical researchers have long known that stress depresses immune function, but only recently have they linked stress to changes in gut bacteria. (See Chapters 2 and 3 for more on how good bacteria help your immune system function properly.)

Collaborating researchers at Ohio State University and Texas Tech University discovered that exposure to stress changes the composition, diversity, and raw numbers of bacteria in the gut. Fewer kinds of good bacteria live in the digestive system of stressed subjects, and harmful bacteria proliferate.

This early research indicates that stress or psychological pressure has a significant impact on gut bacteria populations, which in turn affects immune function. This connection may explain why certain diseases, such as inflammatory bowel disease (see Chapter 4) and asthma, often seem to get worse during periods of unusual stress.

Other research indicates that gut bacteria may play a role in stimulating behavior that benefits immune function. When you're sick, you usually feel sluggish and perhaps even depressed; you don't move as quickly or as much as you do when you're healthy. This lack of physical and mental energy may be an immune system response that helps speed recovery. Studies in mice indicate that certain bacteria have a calming effect on behavior, similar to your own lethargic demeanor during sickness.

Exploring the brain-bacteria link

What if the next generation of antidepressants came in the form of foods like yogurt? Scientists are discovering more every day about the link between your brain chemistry and the bacteria in your gut — and yogurt laced with antidepressant bacteria is one possible therapy that may arise from this research.

To understand how gut bacteria impact brain chemistry, researchers in Ireland fed mice a broth containing *Lactobacillus rhamnosus JB-1*, a strain of good bacteria that lives naturally in your digestive tract. The researchers then compared the mice's behavior and brain chemistry to those of mice that were fed plain broth.

Brain cells have *receptors* that receive and respond to chemical signals from other cells. One of these chemicals, a neurotransmitter called *gamma-aminobutyric acid*, or GABA, inhibits activity in the central nervous system and regulates several physiological and psychological processes in the brain. In people who suffer from depression, certain GABA receptor components are decreased; when you suffer from stress or anxiety, certain GABA receptor components are increased.

In the bacteria-fed mice, the GABA receptor components associated with depression were higher, while the receptor components associated with stress and anxiety were lower. The results indicate that the bacteria helped maintain normal brain chemistry.

In addition, the bacteria-fed mice exhibited much less behavior associated with stress, anxiety, and depression, and levels of stress hormones were significantly lower when the bacteria-fed mice were exposed to stressful situations like mazes.

Just as important as learning that this particular bacteria strain influences the same neurochemicals that antidepressants and anti-anxiety medications target is figuring out how the brain and gut bacteria communicate. The *vagus nerve* connects the brain with the digestive system, and the researchers in this study confirmed that the *Lactobacillus* strain used this same pathway to exchange information with the brain. When researchers cut the vagus nerve in the bacteria-fed mice, the bacteria's impact was lost; neither the mice's behavior nor GABA receptor levels changed.

Changing behavior by changing gut bacteria

Canadian researchers have demonstrated a link between gut bacteria and behavior in mice, which may have implications for treating behavioral disorders in humans.

The researchers used germ-free mice and colonized their digestive tracts with bacteria from mice with different behavioral patterns to see whether the bacteria influenced the mice's behavior. Germ-free mice whose genetic background favored passive behavior were given bacteria from mice with more exploratory behaviors, and genetically active mice were given bacteria from mice with passive backgrounds.

The results of the experiments showed that the different bacteria compositions changed the mice's predicted behavior patterns. Mice with passive genetic backgrounds became more active and daring, while mice with active backgrounds became more passive.

This research indicates that any disruption to the gut bacteria — whether from illness, antibiotics, or other factors — can have a significant impact on behavior. And because certain digestive ailments, such as irritable bowel syndrome, are associated with behavioral disorders, probiotics may have therapeutic potential for restoring normal gut bacteria and alleviating gastrointestinal problems.

One small French study seems to indicate that what happens in mice and rats can happen in humans too. In a 30-day trial, 55 healthy men and women were randomly assigned to take either a daily probiotic supplement consisting of *Lactobacillus helveticus R0052* and *Bifidobacterium longum R0175*, or a placebo. Participants filled out questionnaires before and after treatment to assess their mood, stress levels, and coping skills; in addition, researchers measured stress hormone levels in participants' urine.

Compared with the placebo group, the probiotic group had lower levels of urinary stress hormones and reported less depression, anger, and hostility, and the kind of worry that can lead to physical symptoms.

The research into the connection between probiotics and physical and mental health is both encouraging and exciting. However, all the research to date indicates that only certain specific strains of good bacteria confer these specific health benefits. So don't count on eating today's live-culture yogurts to treat your depression or anxiety symptoms; chances are, the products on the shelves aren't properly formulated for such specific therapeutic uses. Much more research is needed to discover exactly which probiotic strains are most beneficial.

Chapter 2

Looking at Bacterial Behavior in Your Body

*T*he word *bacteria* is enough to send many people scrambling for anti-bacterial hand soap. But bacteria have gotten a bad rap. In fact, good bacteria function throughout your body to keep you healthy. Getting these "good guys" out of whack can make you sick.

Good bacteria can help you digest food, and lots of them are always present in your body. Researchers at the National Human Genome Research project found that each person hosts an average of 1,000 different types of bacteria — just on the *skin*. Clearly, if all bacteria were bad, you'd be losing the battle to stay healthy. Good bacteria even help fight off some of the bad bacteria that cause illness or disease.

One key to bacteria's role in your body is maintaining balance, or keeping the good bacteria at a healthy level. In this chapter, I explore how your digestive system works and how good bacteria help keep you fit and feeling good.

Exploring Your Digestive System

The digestive process starts when you put a bite of food in your mouth. Your saliva immediately goes to work breaking down that tasty morsel into elements your body can use. Your mouth is also loaded with bacteria, mostly the harmless kind. Some bacteria are swallowed and killed by stomach acids, and others may proliferate and cause problems such as tooth decay and gum disease.

Whether you're noshing on a steak, an apple, or a slice of pizza, all the food you eat follows the same path through your digestive system, or *gastrointestinal tract* (often called the *GI tract*): mouth, throat (*pharynx*), esophagus, stomach, small intestine, and large intestine (or *colon*, which includes the rectum). Figure 1-1 shows the human digestive tract.

Your GI tract performs two crucial functions:

✔ Breaking down food to provide nutrients for the body

✔ Preventing harmful substances from being absorbed

When you swallow, the food moves through your digestive system by a process called *peristalsis*. As food comes in contact with the GI tract, muscles contract and propel the food forward, sort of like a wave in the ocean. The esophagus — or food pipe — transports food from the throat to the stomach.

When that chocolate bar or piece of steak enters your stomach, hydrochloric acid and digestive enzymes break it into small particles. *Parietal cells*, located in the lining of your stomach, react to the presence of food and secrete acid to break it down. (Your stomach produces an average of two liters of acid every day.)

After the food is pulverized in the stomach, it's pushed into the small intestine, which is approximately 20 feet long. The small intestine digests food particles, extracting nutrients that your body absorbs. Much of what remains after this process is waste from the body's perspective. After that it enters the colon—the 6-foot large intestine. Water from this waste is absorbed, and the remainder, the fecal matter, is eliminated by bowel movements through the rectum and anus.

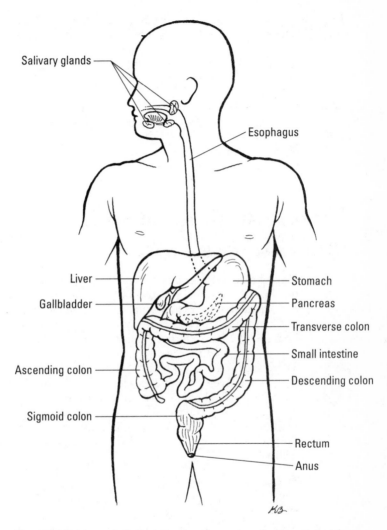

Figure 2-1: Food travels through the digestive system, from mouth to colon.

The colon is lined with the *mucosal barrier*, also called the *epithelial barrier*. The epithelial cells, also called the *colonocytes*, are the gatekeepers of the gut. A healthy mucosal barrier prevents the body from absorbing harmful organisms and toxins. But if the barrier is compromised — for example, overusing antibiotics can wear away spots in the barrier — those weak spots can allow some pretty nasty stuff to get into your bloodstream and wreak all kinds of havoc on your health.

Billions of adherence sites in the intestinal epithelial cells offer places for different bacteria in your gut to grab on. The friendly bacteria overcrowd the bad bacteria by competing for these sites. If the adherence sites are taken, there's no place for the bad bacteria to "stick on."

Your overall health depends on the healthy functioning of your digestive system. Not only does it pull nutrients from food to nourish your body, it also helps protect you against disease. In the following sections, I look at the major role bacteria play in both of these essential functions.

Understanding Good and Bad Bacteria

Bacteria are single-celled microorganisms found everywhere on Earth — in water, soil, plants, and in most parts of your body. In fact, bacteria outnumber the actual cells in your body by about 10 to 1. Your skin and digestive system alone host about 2,000 different kinds of bacteria.

There are fewer bacteria in the stomach than in other parts of the digestive system because its acidic environment kills most bacteria. That makes delivering probiotics particularly challenging — you have to ensure that those good bacteria can survive in the stomach's unfriendly environment. (See Chapter 3 for more on protecting probiotics from stomach acid.)

These organisms acquired their bad reputation in the 1800s, when Louis Pasteur, the father of microbiology, showed that bacterial growth caused spoilage of foods, including milk and beer. He invented the process of heating milk to kill bacteria and mold, now called *pasteurization*. Pasteur proposed that bacteria also cause disease in people, which launched a field that today does much to keep you healthy.

Not all bacteria are bad. In fact, scientists now know that even the "bad" bacteria in your body don't cause problems as long as your system has enough good bacteria to keep them in check. When you're healthy and have the proper bacterial balance in your body, the ratio of good to bad bacteria is about

10 to 1. *Dysbiosis* is the medical term doctors use when this balance is disturbed and the ratio changes. It means you're out of sync between the good, protective bacteria and the harmful, bad bacteria. Even though you have close to 1,000 species of bacteria in your gut, numbering about 100 trillion bacteria, just 30 species make up more than 90 percent of your gut bacteria.

More and more, research is showing that bacterial diversity is an important factor in health and disease. It appears diversity provides resilience. As you age, your bacterial diversity decreases, and this may make you more prone to disease. Decreased bacterial diversity has also been found in obesity (see Chapter 9) and irritable bowel syndrome (see Chapter 4).

In the following sections, I look at the differences between good and bad bacteria and why keeping the proper balance is so important.

Keeping the proper bacterial balance

The bacteria that populate your GI tract are known as *gut microbiota* or *gut flora*. Without these tiny helpers, your body wouldn't be able to absorb vital nutrients or carry out its regular maintenance functions.

Gut flora's nutritional functions include

✔ Producing digestive enzymes that break down food into nutrients the body can use.

✔ Combining various nutrients to generate essential vitamins (a process called *synthesizing)* such as thiamine, folic acid, and vitamin K, among others.

✔ Helping the body absorb nutrients like calcium, iron, and magnesium.

Gut flora also help keep the lining of your GI tract intact and healthy. The cells that line your colon need energy to regenerate themselves; gut flora convert unabsorbed sugars into specific types of fatty acids that your cells use for energy.

Imbalance in the gut flora (friendly versus harmful) can lead to digestive upset that, if left unchecked, can cause far more serious health problems. Research indicates that some people have irritable bowel syndrome because of such an imbalance, for example (see Chapter 4).

Table 1-1 lists some of the most common good and bad bacteria. When good and bad gut flora get out of balance — that is, when bad bacteria proliferate, and you don't have enough good bacteria — you get sick. Symptoms can range from the extremely mild (a general sense of not feeling well or mild diarrhea, for example) to the extremely serious.

Table 1-1	Bacteria: The Good and the Bad
Good bacteria	*Bad bacteria*
Lactobacillus	Salmonella
Bifidobacteria	Shigella
Bacteroides	E. coli
	Clostridium difficile

Seeing how good bacteria work

Gut flora are unique to every individual — almost like fingerprints — beginning at birth and evolving through your life. The GI tract of a human fetus is *sterile,* or completely free of bacteria and fungi. During birth, babies swallow the bacteria present in the birth canal, and within days these bacteria colonize the newborn's intestine. (Babies born via C-section have delayed colonization and may acquire more organisms from the environment, rather than the mother's birth canal, compared to vaginally born infants.)

Your flora fingerprint is established by around the age of 2, and you'll have those same bacteria for the rest of your life. Your body recognizes the bacteria as "normal." Essentially, these bacteria are your colonic warriors: They recognize each other and work to prevent foreign invasion.

Years ago, scientists believed that humans and the bacteria in their bodies had a *commensal* relationship — meaning that

Seventy to 90 percent of your immune system is located in your GI tract, where gut flora work in several ways:

✔ Producing enzymes and proteins that can kill or inhibit harmful bacteria

✔ Crowding out the "bad" bacteria by giving them no space to grab on

✔ Stimulating the secretion of Immunoglobulin A, an antibody that fights infection

Out-of-whack bacterial balances are associated with several illnesses and disorders, from diarrhea to allergies to certain forms of cancer and heart disease. Part II of this book is devoted to more in-depth discussions about the role good bacteria and probiotic supplements play in a variety of health issues.

Gut barrier: Excluding and eliminating harmful elements

The gut barrier is essentially composed of three barriers:

✔ Mechanical barrier (the mucosal epithelial cells)

✔ Ecological barrier (gut bacteria)

✔ Immune barrier (discussed previously)

The epithelium, gut bacteria, and immune cells work together to prevent invasion of potentially harmful substances. The barriers prevent harmful material in the gut's *lumen*, or inside space, from entering the tissues and blood circulatory system.

Discovering How Things Can Go Wrong

Many factors influence the bacteria in your body, in both positive and negative ways. Diet, climate changes, stress, illness, and certain medications can affect the microbiota in your body. Medications such as antibiotics may alter your digestive system's environment, decreasing the number of good bacteria and helping the bad bacteria and fungi (yeast) prolif-erate. *Clostridum difficile* colitis, an infection that causes diar-rhea, and yeast infections are good examples. (See Chapter 4 for more on various forms of diarrhea and Chapter 6 for more on yeast and other types of infections.)

Other acid-reducing medications such as H2 blockers (Zantac and Pepcid) and proton pump inhibitors (omeprazole and Prevacid) can increase the chance of bacterial problems as well. Those meds decrease acid in the stomach and increase the pH, which may allow the bad bacteria to make their way into the colon, causing dysbiosis.

The food you eat has a direct impact on your gut flora. Good bacteria thrive on fresh vegetables (they like the fiber, too), whole grains, and fermented foods like yogurt, kefir, and sau-erkraut. Garlic and green tea are also good for good bacteria. (Check out Chapter 11 for more on probiotic-rich foods and Chapter 12 for probiotic recipes.)

Bad bacteria like animal fats and refined sugars and flours. In addition, dairy and meat products from animals that are treated with antibiotics, steroids, growth hormones, and other drugs can throw the balance between good and bad bacteria out of whack. One study shows that diets rich in meat fat and low in fiber increase the risk of colon cancer (see Chapter 9).

Additives and pesticides, as well as chlorinated water, also can negatively affect your gut flora. Some reports suggest that alcohol and coffee kill good intestinal bacteria, too.

Antibiotics present the greatest known danger to good intes-tinal bacteria. Although antibiotics are quite useful in fighting off many kinds of bacterial infections, these drugs don't dis-tinguish between friendly and harmful bacteria. As a result, a typical course of antibiotic treatment can easily decimate the good bacteria in your GI tract, and it can take four to eight weeks for them to repopulate. Turn to Chapter 4 for more information on antibiotics and gut flora.

Pointing fingers at environmental factors

Along with diet and nutrition, other environmental factors affect your gut bacteria. For example, when you take antibiotics, you can have antibiotic-`associated diarrhea. H2 blockers and proton pump inhibitors (as mentioned previously) also affect the gut's bacteria.

Psychological stress, infections, climate, metabolic stress, and aging all affect the bacteria in your gut.

Age and gut microbiota

Gut flora undergo substantial changes at each end of your life — as an infant and when you're older. It appears there's a decrease in *Lactobacillus* and *Bifidobacterium* species (the good bacteria) as you age, and an increase in *Clostridium* groups and *Enterobacteria* (bad bacteria) at the same time.

At the same time as those bacterial changes occur, you typically see nutritional changes, increased incidence of disease, and a corresponding increase in medication use. All of those things modify the composition of the gut bacteria, making the elderly more susceptible to infections. It's possible that age-related differences in the gut bacteria may be related to disease progression and frailty in the elderly population. That's certainly an area that will receive a lot of research attention in the coming decades.

Chapter 3

Discovering Prebiotics and Probiotics

*G*ood bacteria play a crucial role in maintaining your health and helping you fight disease. Probiotics are supplements of good bacteria, designed to help your body maintain a bacterial balance that will keep you in optimal health.

Natural probiotics — found in food products like kefir and yogurt — have been around for centuries, and many cultures have recognized their healthful properties. But today, evolving diets and longer lives (age tends to shift the bacterial balance in our bodies) mean that most people need supplements to get adequate probiotics.

In this chapter, I explain what prebiotics and probiotics are and how they work together to boost both your digestive health and your general wellbeing. I also look at why it's important to get *both* prebiotics and probiotics in the same supplement and explore how to choose a good supplement for your needs.

Defining the Terms: What Prebiotics and Probiotics Are

The word *probiotics* means "for (or pro) life." In 2001, the World Health Organization (www.who.int) coined the following definition for probiotics:

> *"Probiotics are live microorganisms, which, when administered in adequate amounts, confer a health benefit on the host."*

In other words, probiotics are "good" bacteria. Your intestine's friendly bacteria can be called your *indigenous probiotics*.

Prebiotics are non-digestible food ingredients, like *inulin*, that stimulate the growth and/or activity of good bacteria in the digestive system in ways believed to be beneficial to health.

Looking at the Role of Prebiotics

Scientific understanding of prebiotics — dietary fiber that provides nutrition for probiotics — is relatively new. These fiber food ingredients were first defined in 1995, and the medical community's interest in probiotics has created an interest in prebiotics because their relationship is intertwined.

The standard diet is too often full of processed foods and sugars and low in fiber. This lack of prebiotics affects the efficiency of probiotics.

In the following sections, I talk about what prebiotics do in your digestive system and how they help probiotics do their job.

Understanding what prebiotics are

Prebiotics are food ingredients that pass through your digestive system without being digested by you. They alter the composition or metabolism of the gut microbiota in a beneficial way, serving as food to the good bacteria and helping them flourish.

To be called a prebiotic, a substance should

✔ Be resistant to gastric acidity and host enzymes — that is, not digestible by the host.

✔ Be fermented by gut microbiota.

✔ Stimulate growth and activity of the gut flora microbiota, which contributes to your health and wellbeing.

When you ingest prebiotic fiber, the fermentation that takes place in your gut helps with water and electrolyte reabsorption and produces *short chain fatty acids* (SCFAs), which help maintain the lining of the bowel (see Chapter 1). Fiber can be *water insoluble* or *water soluble*. Bacteria in the gut ferment less than 50 percent of water-insoluble fiber, whereas water-soluble fiber is fermented well by your gut microbiota.

Here are some common foods that contain prebiotics:

✔ Artichokes

✔ Bananas

✔ Barley

✔ Chicory

✔ Flax

✔ Garlic

✔ Oats

✔ Onions

✔ Soybeans and soybean products such as tofu

✔ Wheat

How prebiotics work

Prebiotic fiber is fermented by gut microbiota, creating short chain fatty acids, the primary ones being *acetate propionate* and *butyrate*. SCFAs help you in many ways, including producing energy by working as a fuel source for your colon's *epithelium* (the cells lining the inside of your colon), helping with electrolyte and water absorption and modulating immune function.

In addition to being an energy source, prebiotics seem to act as a stimulus for the bacterial epithelial "cross talk" or communication (as described in Chapter 2). Some prebiotics can also prevent pathogenic "bad" bacteria from adhering to the colons epithelial cells. For example, *oligofructose* can interfere with the receptors of pathogenic bacteria by binding tightly to them and preventing them from attaching to the colon's epithelium. When bad bacteria can't adhere, it's more difficult for them to cause you harm.

Other research, still in early stages, indicates that prebiotics can directly stimulate the immune system. It seems that SCFAs, especially *butyrate*, decrease the incidence of inflammatory bowel disease and colon cancer. (Find more on those conditions in Chapter 4 and 9, respectively.)

Understanding the Functions of Probiotics

Probiotics perform useful functions when you ingest them. For example, probiotics produce vitamins, especially the B vitamins and vitamin K2. Vitamin K is essential for blood clotting; vitamin K1 is of plant origin, and vitamin K2 is made by gut bacteria. B-complex vitamins produced by probiotics include biotin, thiamine, pantothenic acid, pyridoxine, folic acid, and vitamin B12. These all play a key role in energy metabolism.

In the following sections, I outline a number of probiotics' beneficial effects. These benefits include helping the immune system, providing protection against "bad" bacteria, and improving both digestive function and your general health.

Boosting the immune system

The immune system protects the body against intruding microbes and environmental agents. It's a dynamic network of proteins, organs, cells, and tissues (see Chapter 2).

Many researchers are exploring how probiotics work at the molecular and genetic levels, and ample evidence shows that probiotics boost the immune system.

One way probiotics boost immunity is by increasing the production of *mucin*, proteins that are found in saliva and the mucosal linings of your gastrointestinal tract. Mucin helps protect against friction and erosion and also creates an unfavorable environment for bad bacteria.

Evidence shows that probiotics boost immunity in people with sub-optimal immune systems, such as the elderly or people in stressful situations. Probiotics also stimulate the immune system in other situations where immunity and inflammatory responses are out of control — for example, in autoimmune diseases such as rheumatoid arthritis. Probiotics seem to encourage *immunomodulation*, the balance of control between pro-inflammatory and anti-inflammatory cytokines. *Cytokines* are substances secreted by your immune system that affect other cells.

Research has shown that probiotics have a number of effects on the immune system, depending on what your body needs. Probiotics

✔ Increase production of *immunoglobulin A* (IgA) *antibodies*, proteins that recognize and fight foreign invaders in your body. (See Chapter 8 for more on different types of antibodies.)

✔ Decrease the number of *inflammatory mediators*, molecules that immune cells release when you have an infection. Lower numbers of these molecules suggest that probiotics help heal inflammation.

✔ Decrease production of allergy-specific *IgE antibodies,* found in lungs, skin, and mucous membranes, causing the body to fight foreign substances like pollen, animal dander, and fungal spores.

Certain probiotic bacteria elicit anti-inflammatory responses in intestinal epithelial cells (see Chapter 2). Probiotics also help maintain and strengthen the gut's defensive barrier.

Protecting the gut's lining

The *gut barrier* is a complex system responsible for your health and includes the gut microbiota, gut mucosa, and your immune system.

In addition to the gut barrier, you have what's called a "non-specific" barrier in the *lumen* (the hollow part of the gut), which includes gastric acid, mucus digestive enzymes, and *peristal*sis (a wavelike movement in the digestive tract), which prevents bacteria from entering your bloodstream. When the gut barrier breaks down (because of digestive illness or other illness that disrupts the barrier), *intestinal permeability* increases, allowing harmful bacteria and other substances to enter your bloodstream. Such changes in intestinal permeability, commonly called "leaky gut," may be responsible for conditions such as inflammatory bowel disease, cancer, and, in some patients, irritable bowel syndrome.

The epithelial cells that line the colon are part of the mucosal barrier that prevents the body from absorbing harmful organisms and toxins. These cells have adherence sites, and the probiotic bacteria stick to them, leaving no place for the harmful bacteria to attach. See Chapter 2 for more on the digestive system's anatomy.

Many probiotics release antibacterial substances called *bacteriocins* that selectively reduce the growth of bad bacteria. In addition, many probiotics produce other substances, such as lactic acid, which help acidify the bowel and prevent harmful bacteria from growing.

Improving digestive health

As the U.S. medical community explores the usefulness of probiotics, the most studied medical area is digestive health, and research clearly shows that probiotics improve digestive health and are beneficial for a host of digestive conditions. Turn to Chapter 4 to explore how probiotics help in a variety of digestive disorders, from irritable bowel syndrome to possibly Crohn's disease.

Although the probiotic role in preventing and curing disease is crucial, the role of generally improving your digestive health is just as critical. Your daily life can have a negative impact on your gut flora. Changes in your gut flora occur as you age, as you take medicine, and as you eat a diet high in meats and fats, among other things.

Probiotics can rebalance the good bacteria in your digestive system, keeping you in tip-top shape to fight off illness and feel your best.

Promoting general health and wellbeing

As I mention elsewhere, the concept of probiotics is an old one, dating to times when people understood the benefits of fermented foods, but didn't have the scientific terms to explain them. Today, researchers are finding hard science support for the folk remedy.

The benefits of probiotics don't stop with the digestive tract. Researchers are continually highlighting the benefits of pro-biotics in other parts of your body, which can impact your overall health and wellbeing.

Even if you're in perfect health, taking probiotics daily helps you maintain the proper balance of bacterial flora in your GI tract. Environmental, dietary, and emotional stressors impact your body, causing changes in your gut flora and other areas of your body. Taking probiotics helps keep the good bacteria in control.

Even more exciting, though, is that probiotics seem to hold great promise for alleviating a broad range of health issues. For example, probiotics may offer options to people strug-gling with health issues ranging from obesity (see Chapters 7 and 8) to allergies (see Chapter 5) to urogenital infections (see Chapter 6). In fact, researchers are investigating the intriguing possibilities of using probiotics to help prevent debilitating conditions such as cancer and heart disease (turn to Chapter 9 to discover more).

Seeing How Prebiotics and Probiotics Work Together

Probiotics and prebiotics work together to maintain gut health in different ways. To get the full benefits of both, so-called *synbiotics* combine them. The three most common pre-biotics are *inulin*, *oligofructose*, and *polydextrose*. When you shop for probiotic supplements, look for these prebiotics on the label.

In the following sections, I explore why your body needs the fiber that prebiotics provide, as well as how combining probiotics and prebiotics enhances the beneficial effects of good bacteria.

Understanding why your body needs fiber

Dietary fiber, also known as roughage or bulk, is usually found in fruits, vegetables, whole grains, and legumes. Your body doesn't digest fiber; humans don't have the machinery to break it down. But your gut bacteria can and do use fiber for energy.

Fiber is classified as either insoluble or soluble, based on whether it dissolves in water. *Insoluble* fiber increases stool bulk and helps with constipation by regularizing bowel movements. Examples of insoluble fiber include whole wheat flour, wheat bran, nuts, and some vegetables, such as green beans, zucchini, and celery.

Soluble fiber absorbs water and becomes a jellylike mass that slows digestion. It lowers cholesterol and glucose levels. Soluble fiber is found in oats, beans, peas, citrus fruits, apples, carrots, barley, and psyllium (a common ingredient in high-fiber cereals), among many other plant foods.

A high-fiber diet, in addition to helping increase bulk, has the following benefits. It

- Increases intestinal transit time and keeps bowel movements normal.

- Maintains bowel health and integrity by decreasing the risk of *diverticulosis*, pouches in the large intestine or colon that bulge outward.

- Decreases risk of hemorrhoids.

- Lowers cholesterol levels.

- Helps control blood sugar levels.

- Aids in weight loss (fewer calories for the same volume of food).

✔ Produces more SCFAs from prebiotic fibers (see "Understanding what prebiotics are" earlier in this chapter).

Looking at synbiotics

The combination of a probiotic and a prebiotic in a single package means the probiotic bacteria will have food. Such combining extends the product's shelf life, as probiotics by themselves may deteriorate on store shelves.

Not only do the prebiotics help the probiotics they're packaged with, but they also feed the indigenous bacteria in your gut. A synbiotic gives you a total package of the probiotics and the food they need to survive and thrive.

Although you can get your prebiotics through foods, the standard American diet — full of processed foods, high in sugar, and low in fiber — doesn't typically provide enough prebiotics to help the good bacteria in your digestive system. So look for prebiotics in your probiotic supplement. Common prebiotics are *inulin* and *oligofructose*. Other prebiotics to look for include *fructooligosaccharides (FOS)*, *galactooligosaccharides (GOS)*, *xylooligosaccharides (XOS)*, *lactulose*, and *polydextrose*.

Probulin (www.probulin.com) is a good example of a synbiotic, where the two elements, probiotics and prebiotics, work together as a one-two boost to your system.

Exploring the Ideal Probiotic

Aggressive marketing by the yogurt and probiotic industries is informing consumers about the benefits of taking probiotic and prebiotic supplements. It's likely just a matter of time before people take such supplements just as they do vitamins and fish oil.

As you add probiotics and prebiotics to your health regimen, consider several factors when choosing an ideal supplement or food product. Ideal probiotics

✔ Are of human (not animal) origin.

✔ Resist acid and bile in the upper GI tract.

✔ Attach to human epithelial cells.

✔ Colonize the intestine.

✔ Produce antimicrobial substances such as enzymes and proteins that fight off bad bacteria.

✔ Boost the immune system.

✔ Are safe in food and for clinical use.

✔ Are documented in clinical studies to be beneficial.

All probiotic products are not the same. You need to look at a host of factors before deciding on a probiotic supplement or product. In the following sections, you discover what you need to know to choose a good probiotic supplement.

Considering genus, species, and strain

Bacteria are identified by their genus and species. The genus is the collection or group in which the bacteria belong; the species is the individual bacteria type.

Some bacteria also have several strains, or variations, within the same species. The name of the strain is attached to the end of the bacteria's formal name. For example, *Lactobacillus acidophilus DDS-1* belongs to the genus *Lactobacillus* and the species *acidophilus*, and *DDS-1* is the specific strain.

When researchers study bacteria and probiotics, they typically study a single strain to determine whether that particular kind of bacterium is useful for a certain health condition. Do your research online or talk to your doctor about which strains of bacteria have been successful in treating your specific health condition.

Because different bacteria target different health issues, it makes sense to take a probiotic that includes several strains of bacteria. In addition, your gut contains 1,000 different types of bacteria, which adds to the logic that having a variety of strains in your supplement is a good idea. Good probiotics usually include *Lactobacillus acidophilus*, *Bifidobacteria,* and at least two or three other bacteria.

Combating gastric acidity

Stomach acid attacks and destroys many bacteria that enter your digestive system, whether they arrive in food or in a pro-biotic supplement. Good probiotics use technology to protect the bacteria from stomach acids. The highest quality probiot-ics are tested in a "simulated acid environment" to make sure the capsule survives the challenging stomach environment.

Probulin is a good example of an acid-protected probiotic. Probulin is made with a proprietary process that minimizes the loss of bacteria to the harsh stomach acid; the probiotics are not released until after the capsule leaves the stomach.

Sticking to it: Adherence and persistence

The property of probiotic bacteria that makes them "stick to" the epithelial cells of the colonic mucosa is called *adherence*. There are billions of sites on the epithelial cells to which good bacteria adhere, and in doing so they prevent the bad bacte-ria from latching on.

Adherence is considered important for stimulation of the immune system. Some bacteria adhere better than others, and the bacteria that do so tend to colonize better. A combina-tion of specific probiotic strains may enhance adherence in a synergistic manner. This is an area of intense research and competition by pharmaceutical companies as they rush to determine which bacteria adhere the best.

Recently, researchers in Ireland have discovered small appendages in *Bifidobacteria* that may help explain how probiotics colonize the intestine. Apparently, *Bifidobacteria* produce finger-like tentacles, called *TAD-pili* (or *pili* for short), that allow them to stick to the gut lining and form colonies. The researchers were able to demonstrate the pili only when the *Bifidobacteria* were in host organisms. The appendages didn't appear when the bacteria were grown in a lab, so apparently they receive a signal from the host to "turn on" the pili.

Persistence describes the ability of the probiotic to implant and survive in the colon long after supplementation. Probiotics that do persist are like gifts that keep on giving. Unfortunately, researchers estimate that 95 percent of the probiotics in supplements today lack the property of persistence.

Manufacturing processes and storage methods

Manufacturing processes and storage methods are critical to probiotics' efficacy. Manufacturers use different stabilizers to prevent loss of bacteria during shipping and storage. Obviously, a well-formulated product maintains stability during those critical steps from the manufacturing plant to your store shelves.

Some probiotic products contain far fewer bacteria than listed on their labels. While that's a challenge for you as a consumer, because it's difficult to know which labels are accurate, being cognizant of how a product is manufactured is important. During manufacturing, shipping, and storage, bacterial concentration can shift. Today, many websites contain detailed information on their products, so, with a little effort, you may be able to determine which companies are careful in their handling practices.

After you buy your probiotic supplement, read the label carefully, as some probiotics may need to be refrigerated. Even if the package doesn't indicate the need for refrigeration, always store your probiotics in a cool place. Most probiotics are stable for several months as long as they're not exposed to heat and moisture. Research shows that moisture reduces the lifespan of probiotics.

When bacteria are frozen or dried during the manufacturing process, they become dormant and enter a state of suspended animation. That means they're still alive, but basically "frozen" in time. When the bacteria are exposed to moisture, they come out of the "cocoon" and become active again. That's why it is important to keep your probiotics dry; you don't want the bacteria to become active in your bathroom cabinet.

Bacteria have been reported to survive in suspended animation for 4,800 years in the stonework of the Peruvian pyramids. But these days those bacteria seem young, as scientists have discovered 34,000-year-old bacteria living in Death Valley salt crystals.

Looking at labeling standards

Although the U.S. Food and Drug Administration regulates labeling for dietary supplements and reviews ingredients for safety (not effectiveness), the agency does not endorse or approve any dietary supplements. Several independent organizations, including Consumerlab.com, NSF International (www.nsf.org), and U.S. Pharmacopeia (www.usp.org), allow manufacturers to display seals on their labels if they pass tests for quality, manufacturing processes, and other standards.

A good probiotic label should have

- A list of all bacteria in the product.
- The number of colony forming units (CFUs) of bacteria. The more CFUs, the better; look for products with 1 to 10 billion CFUs.
- An expiration date or suggested final date of use.
- A listing of any other ingredients (for example, the prebiotic *inulin*).

What to Expect When You Start Taking Probiotics

When you start taking probiotic supplements, you may experience an increase in gas and bloating. These symptoms usually disappear within a week, and most people begin to notice a better sense of physical wellbeing after the initial effects wear off.

Your experience when you begin taking probiotics may differ, depending on your reasons for taking them. For example, if you get acute diarrhea while traveling, taking probiotics means you get over the diarrhea faster. If you're taking anti-biotics for an infection, there is a decreased chance you'll get antibiotic-associated diarrhea if you take probiotics at the same time.

With more chronic bowel problems, taking probiotics improves bowel function, and most people will see an improvement within two weeks.

Probiotics belong to the "Generally Recognized as Safe" (GRAS) category as compiled by the U.S. Food and Drug Administration (www.fda.gov). The GRAS designation means that experts consider these food additives — chemicals, pre-servatives, or other substances — to be safe for human con-sumption. Probiotics are considered so safe that they are now routinely added to infant formulas.

Part II

Preserving and Improving Health with Probiotics

The 5th Wave   By Rich Tennant

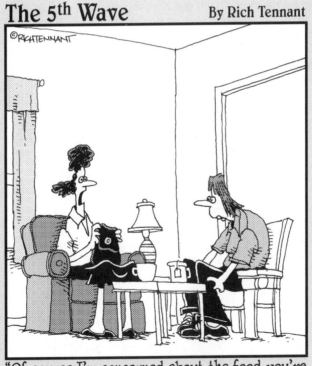

"Of course I'm concerned about the food you're serving your family. Let's face it, you named your first three children Twinkie, Ding Dong, and Fluffernutter."

In this part . . .

*N*ow that you have an understanding of how bacteria work in your body and how probiotics — the good bacteria — can help, let's explore the different systems in your body and look at what research is finding out about helpful bacteria. The most well-studied area is the gut so I start there, showing how probiotics have been effective in treating many intestinal diseases and illnesses. But probiotics aren't just for your gut, and in this part I also investigate the implications for other health challenges, including urogenital problems such as yeast and urinary tract infections, as well as some of the promising probiotics research into treating such varied conditions as cancer, diabetes, and rheumatoid arthritis.

Chapter 4

Starting with the Obvious: Digestive Health

*T*he health of your digestive system is crucial to your overall feeling of wellbeing and to maintaining your body at its optimum function. Your digestive system is influenced by many factors, including the foods you eat, the bacteria you come in contact with, and the way your body changes as you age.

In the past 20 years, we've advanced our understanding of what probiotics are and how they help your digestive system. Probiotics are an important part of maintaining digestive health, supplementing the good bacteria already in your system, fighting bad bacteria, and preventing disease. Consumer and physician awareness of probiotics has been increasing exponentially. It's clear today that probiotics play a key role in not only preserving and improving digestive health, but also in preventing certain digestive diseases.

Considering the Use of Antibiotics

The ancient Egyptians, Chinese, and Central American Indians used mold to treat infections, so they are credited with using the first anti-bacterial treatment. Antibiotics — a word derived from the Greek *anti* meaning against, and *bios* meaning life — were developed in the late 1800s when medical science began to accept the *germ theory of disease* (the idea that bacteria and other microbes cause disease). This theory was highly controversial when it was first proposed, but, once validated, it became the cornerstone of modern medicine and led to important innovations such as antibiotics.

Understanding how antibiotics work

The first effective antibiotic was penicillin, discovered in the 1920s by Sir Alexander Fleming. (Two German doctors, Rudolf Emmerich and Oscar Low, first used an antibiotic in the 1880s, called *pyocyanase*, but it often wasn't effective.) Today, numerous antibiotics work in two ways:

✔ *Bactericidal* antibiotics kill bacteria.

✔ *Bacteriostatic* antibiotics stop bacteria from multiplying.

Antibiotics are ineffective against viruses, so they are not used to treat viral illnesses, such as the common cold.

Exploring antibiotics

Doctors prescribe antibiotics for infections caused by bacteria, fungi, and parasites. Different antibiotics work best in specific situations. Depending on the severity and site of the infection, your doctor may prescribe antibiotics orally or, for more severe infections, intravenously. Antibiotics can be given topically also for localized skin infections or as drops for eye or ear infections.

Antibiotics work in various ways, with some targeting bacterial function and others impacting the organism's physical structure.

Penicillins and cephalosporins attack the cell wall. Polymyxins attack the cell membrane. Quinilones (such as Cipro and Levaquin) and sulfonamides interfere with the essential bacterial enzymes. Tetracyclines and aminoglycosides attack protein synthesis in bacteria. Broad-spectrum antibiotics attack several different types of bacteria, while narrow-spectrum antibiotics target specific bacteria.

Following the evolution of antibiotics

The first antibiotics, penicillin and streptomycin, treated certain illnesses or diseases. They were considered narrow-spectrum antibiotics that targeted specific bacteria. Doctors wanted antibiotics that would treat a range of infections, and in the 1940s labs were successful in finding broad-spectrum antibiotics. In the 1950s, tetracycline was introduced and became the most prescribed broad-spectrum antibiotic in the United States.

Looking at the dark side of antibiotics

Antibiotics have saved thousands of lives, but they also can cause problems. Side effects, minor or major, are not unusual. Minor problems include nausea and skin rashes. Major problems include anaphylaxis (a life-threatening allergic reaction), kidney failure, diarrhea, and vaginal yeast infections.

Antibiotic resistance is a critical concern. Overuse of antibiotics — or using them incorrectly, such as stopping their use prematurely — can cause bacteria to become resistant to the antibiotics.

This antibiotic resistance is one of the biggest concerns in medicine today. Antibiotic-resistant bacteria can cause infections that can't be treated. An example is MRSA, or Methicillin-resistant *Staphylococcus aureus*. This superbug came about after doctors started to treat staph infections with Methicillin, an antibiotic closely related to penicillin. Over time, bacteria developed that resisted the antibiotic, creating the superbug that today causes serious medical complications.

Many patients fail to take antibiotics appropriately, adding to the problem of antibiotic resistance. If you don't finish your prescription of antibiotics and fully get rid of your illness, then the bacteria may recover and become resistant to the antibiotics. The old saying "whatever doesn't kill me only makes me stronger" is applicable to bacteria.

In addition to resistance issues, antibiotics may have side effects, including soft stools, diarrhea, or mild stomach upset. More serious side effects can be vomiting, severe watery diarrhea, abdominal cramps, and allergic reactions.

Doing the Potty Dance: Probiotics and Diarrhea

You've probably experienced the frantic rush for a bathroom, legs crossed and teeth gritted. Usually diarrhea is associated with a gastrointestinal (GI) illness, or possibly food you've eaten. The word *diarrhea* comes from a Greek word meaning "flowing through" — a perfectly accurate summary of those loose, watery, and frequent stools.

You may accept diarrhea as a relatively ordinary thing, but it can be serious. It's one of the most common causes of death in the world — especially in developing countries, where it causes dehydration and electrolyte imbalance.

Acute diarrhea is of short duration, and *chronic* diarrhea is of long duration. The acute type is often caused by infections, such as viral rotavirus in children and norovirus in adults, or from bacterial-related infections like campylobacter, *E.coli*, salmonella, or shigella. It also can result from using antibiotics (*C. difficile* diarrhea).

Occasionally, acute diarrhea causes severe illness, requiring immediate medical attention. It can cause fever, dysentery (bloody, mucusy diarrhea), and dehydration. Most cases improve with oral hydration (water, sports drinks, fruit juice, broth, and so on), although serious cases may require intravenous fluids.

Chronic diarrhea can be caused by

- Irritable bowel syndrome (IBS).
- Inflammatory bowel disease (IBD), including Crohn's disease and ulcerative colitis.
- Lactose intolerance.
- Malabsorption (caused by pancreatic problems or bowel problems such as celiac disease).

✔ Chronic alcoholism.

✔ Parasitic infections like giardiasis and amoebiasis.

✔ Drugs.

✔ Hyperthyroidism.

✔ Colon cancer.

✔ Radiation.

Probiotics have been used by physicians and consumers for diarrhea for several years. Ample anecdotal evidence (backed by research in some instances) indicates probiotics help alleviate diarrhea of various causes.

In 2006, a national panel of experts recommended that probiotics be used for anyone with antibiotic-related diarrhea and acute diarrhea. That panel also said probiotics hold promise for IBS and IBD, as discussed later in this chapter.

Fighting an epidemic: C. difficile diarrhea

It's not uncommon to get diarrhea after taking antibiotics. Most of the time it resolves by itself, or with symptomatic treatment.

Antibiotics tend to decrease or "wipe out" the good bacteria, allowing bad bacteria normally present in small quantities to proliferate. One such bad bacteria is *Clostridium difficile*, commonly called *C. diff.*

C. diff. diarrhea is also called pseudomembranous colitis because of how the colon looks during an endoscopy. It is inflamed and covered with pseudomembranes, or plaque. *C. diff.* causes colitis by producing toxin A and toxin B in the colonic lumen.

C. diff. diarrhea is a classic example of a bacterial imbalance getting you in trouble. The epithelial barrier (see Chapter 2) is compromised, allowing the toxins/bacteria to enter your body and decreasing your immune defenses.

The incidence and severity of *C. diff.* have been increasing in epidemic proportion over the last decade, and so have deaths associated with it. Hypervirulent strains of *C. diff.* throughout North America and Europe have contributed to the epidemic.

C. diff. infections can spread easily from one person to another, especially in a nursing home or hospital setting if the staff doesn't take adequate precautions in terms of cleaning toilets and other surfaces. *C. diff.* bacterial spores can survive on surfaces for a few days and are resistant to several cleansing solutions. Because of these challenges, you can get *C. diff.* even when you haven't been on antibiotics. If you're in the hospital for over four weeks, the chance of getting *C. diff.* is over 50 percent. The annual financial burden of *C. diff.* in the U.S. is estimated to be over a billion dollars.

In spite of treatment, it's recurrent in some individuals, and probiotics are particularly helpful in this situation. In a hospital or nursing home setting, wearing gloves and hand washing with soap and water decreases the incidence of *C. diff.* infection spreading among patients. The increasing use of proton pump inhibiting medications (such as omeprazole) for acid reflux disease or peptic ulcer disease is partly responsible for the increase in *C. diff.* diarrhea. The stomach is a highly acidic environment because of the hydrochloric acid produced there — a defense mechanism against bad bacteria. Lowering the stomach acid lowers the barrier against these bacteria, creating a higher chance of patients on proton pump inhibitors getting *C. diff.*

C. diff. varies from mild to severe, and is even life-threatening in some cases. You can't take this bacterial infection lightly: It is estimated that 15,000 to 30,000 people die each year from severe *C. diff.* infection in the U.S.

Symptoms include abdominal pain, bloating, diarrhea, fever, and in severe cases bloody diarrhea. Toxins produced by the bacteria cause these symptoms. Diagnosis is made by doing a stool test that looks for the toxin that *C. diff.* produces (called clostridium difficile toxin assay, or CDTA). If the test isn't definitive, or the doctor needs to know the severity of the infection, a colonoscopy may be done.

Historically, it's been customary to recommend that patients eat yogurt when they take antibiotics, and many doctors are beginning to prescribe probiotics along with antibiotics. Pediatricians have been among the first to recognize the validity of this practice, and have been moving quickly to prescribe the two together. The research is certainly out there to back up the idea that taking a probiotic when you take an antibiotic decreases the chance you'll get a *C. diff.* infection. With rising occurrences of *C. diff.*, it's likely the rest of the medical profession will soon follow suit.

Looking at standard medical treatments

If you have a *C. diff.* infection, the first thing your doctor will do is stop the antibiotic you are taking. Then you're typically given one of three drugs — metranidazole (Flagyl), vancomycin (Vancocin), or rifaximin (Xifaxan) — to treat *C. difficile* infections. It's been shown that taking probiotics for 30 days along with these medicines decreases the number of days of diarrhea and recurrence of the infection. Occasionally patients with severe *C. diff.* may continue to get worse in spite of treatment and may need a colectomy (removal of the colon).

Another option that causes many people to shudder in disgust is fecal bacteriotherapy, also called stool transplantation. Physicians in Australia have transplanted stool from normal, healthy family donors into patients who are very sick with *C. diff.* and have had good results saving patient lives. Only a few centers in the U.S. have used this treatment on severely ill patients. The rationale is to reintroduce normal flora into the sick patient's colon, overcoming the *C. diff.* bacteria and restoring colon *homeostasis*, the healthy balance between good and bad bacteria. Even though the concept is aesthetically unpleasant and disgusting, it could save your life one day. In the near future, it's possible we'll see a surge of probiotic enemas to treat *C. diff.*, a procedure that would use the same rationale as bacteriotherapy.

Using probiotics for C. difficile diarrhea

Lactobacillus rhamnosus GG and *Lactobacillus acidophilus* have shown promise in treatment of *C. diff.* and prevention of recurrences. Those are the two probiotics typically prescribed by doctors along with antibiotics. The probiotic yeast *Saccharomyces boulardii* has also shown some promise, primarily in treatment of recurrent *C. diff.* infections. In one study, the use of the antibiotic vancomycin along with the probiotics yeast *Saccharomyces boulardii* achieved a higher cure rate than vancomycin alone. It appears that the yeast produces a protease (an enzyme) that inactivates *C. diff.* toxin A.

Looking at other types of diarrhea

Infectious or contagious diarrhea (a category that encompasses viral or bacterial gastroenteritis) can be caused by the following:

- Viruses (rotavirus in children; others include norovirus, adenovirus, astrovirus)
- Bacteria (*Campylobacter jejuni, Salmonella, Shigella, E. coli, C. diff.*)
- Toxins of bacteria (Staphylococcal toxins)
- Parasites (*Giardia lamblia, Entamoeba histolytica*)
- Worms (hookworm, pinworm, tapeworm; mostly in developing countries, rare in the U.S.)

Since 2000, the rotavirus vaccine has helped to decrease the number of infectious diarrhea cases caused by the rotavirus. Typically, doctors treat such infections symptomatically with fluids and, if a stool test identifies the cause as bacterial, with appropriate antibiotic treatment.

The role of probiotics is being defined by more research every year. Studies in kids with viral gastroenteritis show that probiotics reduce the duration of the symptoms.

Gastroenteritis

Gastroenteritis — also called gastric flu, stomach flu, or stomach virus — is a severe inflammation of the GI tract. It often causes nausea, abdominal pain, vomiting, and diarrhea. It can be transferred by contact with food or water.

The causes of gastroenteritis can be viral, including norovirus, rotavirus, adenovirus, and astrovirus, and bacterial, caused by *Salmonella, Shigella, Campylobacteria, E. coli, Yersinia, Vibrio cholerae*, and others. Occasionally, parasites like *Giardia* can cause the illness. You also can get dysentery with bacterial gastroenteritis.

Treatment for gastroenteritis tends to be *symptomatic* (the symptoms are treated). It's important to get anyone with gastroenteritis hydrated, because they can become dehydrated rapidly. Antibiotics may be given if the root cause is determined to be bacterial with stool tests.

Probiotics have been shown to be beneficial in preventing and treating various forms of gastroenteritis. Research has shown that probiotics reduce both the duration of the illness and the frequency of the diarrhea. Fermented milk products such as yogurt or kefir also reduce the duration of symptoms.

Probiotics studied for use in treating/preventing gastroenteritis include *Lactobacillus GG*, *Bifidobacterium bifidum*, *Streptococcus thermophilus*, *Lactobacillus reuteri*, and *Saccharomyces boulardii*.

Traveler's diarrhea

One of the least pleasurable aspects of visiting other countries is traveler's diarrhea (TD), a condition estimated to impact around 10 million Americans each year. TD is defined as three or more stools in a 24-hour period when you are travelling outside of the U.S. It is usually associated with abdominal cramping, bloating, and occasionally nausea. The source of infection is usually ingestion of fecal-contaminated food or water. Men and women get TD at about the same rate, but people at higher risk include young adults and those who are

- ✔ Immunosuppressed.
- ✔ Have irritable bowel disease.
- ✔ Taking acid suppressant medications.
- ✔ Diabetic.

The most common organism to cause TD is *Enterotoxigenic Escherichia coli* (*E. coli*). Other bacteria, parasites, and viruses have also been found to be causative agents.

In addition to diarrhea, you may develop nausea, vomiting, abdominal cramping, fever, urgency, weakness, malaise, decreased appetite, and dehydration.

TD is usually self-limiting and resolves in three or four days, but around 10–20 percent of cases may take a week. Patients occasionally need hospitalization, primarily for dehydration.

Most travelers learn to prevent TD by avoiding local water and ice. If you drink only sealed bottled water and make sure everything you eat is well-cooked, you can often prevent the initial occurrence. Bismuth subsalicylate, found in products such as Pepto-Bismol, has been shown to reduce the incidence of traveler's diarrhea.

Once you get it, drink plenty of fluids and consult a doctor because some patients may need antibiotics and IV fluids. Persistent symptoms may call for stool tests. It's okay to take Immodium or Lomotil to reduce symptoms.

Before taking a trip overseas, start eating yogurt/kefir or begin probiotics a few days before departure. Several probiotics (including *Saccharomyces boulardii* and *Lactobacillus acidophilus*) have been shown to be effective in preventing traveler's diarrhea.

Understanding Inflammatory Bowel Disease (IBD)

Inflammatory bowel disease, or IBD, is a term used to describe a group of autoimmune inflammatory conditions of the GI tract. You may have heard of ulcerative colitis or Crohn's disease, both of which are common inflammatory bowel diseases. Over 1 million Americans suffer from IBD.

Ulcerative colitis and Crohn's disease

Ulcerative colitis affects the colon, with inflammation limited to the mucosa only — the innermost layer of the colon.

Crohn's disease affects the colon and/or the small bowel primarily, but can affect any area of the digestive tract. In Crohn's, the inflammation affects the entire thickness of the intestinal wall.

Exploring symptoms, signs, diagnosis, and treatment

For the most part, symptoms in both of these diseases are very similar. They consist of abdominal pain, diarrhea, weight loss, rectal bleeding, and anemia. Crohn's disease can also cause fistulas around the anus or on the anterior abdominal wall. Patients with either of these two IBDs are at a higher risk of developing colon cancer and will need periodic colonoscopies. Both conditions can go into remission with appropriate treatment.

At age 50, everyone, regardless of symptoms, needs a screening colonoscopy!

Diagnosis is usually made by one or a combination of the following tests: colonoscopy or small bowel X-ray; small bowel capsule endoscopy (where the doctor uses a small camera to get pictures of the small bowel); and a computed tomography (CT) scan of the abdomen.

Currently, the mainstay of treatment for both ulcerative colitis and Crohn's disease is 5-aminosalicylates, which are anti-inflammatory agents. For acute flare-ups, doctors may use short-term steroids. In addition, if the disease can't be controlled, immunosuppressants such as azathioprine can be used. If you have Crohn's with fistulas, metronidazole may be added. More recently, immune modulators have been introduced to treat both diseases (including infliximab, adalimumab, certolizumab). If infection is suspected, antibiotics can be used, and occasionally surgery is an option.

Seeing how probiotics can help

Studies have shown that probiotics can help prevent and treat inflammatory bowel disease. Several have shown show the benefit of probiotics in prolonging the remission period in IBD.

People with IBD have a decreased number of indigenous probiotics, or friendly bacteria, in the colon. That's true even when the IBD is in remission — the situation is worse when the IBD is active. Initial studies have shown a positive role for probiotics for ulcerative colitis, but proof for the effectiveness of probiotics in helping patients with Crohn's disease is unclear. It has been shown that patients with IBD have an alteration in their short-chain fatty acids pattern. Studies showed that SCFA butyrate (see Chapter 3) enemas for six weeks in patients with ulcerative colitis, who were unresponsive to standard therapy, improved their disease state.

At this point in the medical landscape, it seems that probiotics will have a role in treating IBD patients along with traditional treatments. Several trials are underway to determine which probiotics are the most beneficial.

Discovering the Mechanisms of Irritable Bowel Syndrome

Irritable bowel syndrome (IBS) — also called spastic colon, irritable colon, and sensitive gut — is the most common chronic medical condition in the Western world. It's estimated that 15 to 30 million people in the United States have IBS. IBS can cause disruption of life and decreased productivity and is a major cause of work absenteeism.

Defining IBS

In IBS, the gut lining is always normal, unlike in IBD. The symptoms may be so debilitating that around 40 percent of patients with IBS have to take time off work and curtail their social life. IBS is a true disease of the gut and not a "mental condition," as some patients and even physicians believe.

IBS is not psychological! Although stress can aggravate IBS, it is a gut problem, not a psychogenic problem.

Diagnosing IBS

Symptoms of IBS include a combination of the following:

- ✔ Constipation
- ✔ Diarrhea
- ✔ Bloating

> ✔ Abdominal pain
>
> ✔ Gas
>
> ✔ Urgency to go to the bathroom

IBS is divided into three categories: constipation predominant; diarrhea predominant; and alternators, or patients who fluctuate between constipation and diarrhea.

IBS is usually a diagnosis of exclusion, meaning your gastroenterologist will make sure that there is nothing more serious going on in your digestive system (such as IBD or colon cancer) by doing appropriate testing. IBS symptoms may include abdominal pain (cramping or bloating) associated with change in bowel habits. You may have constipation or diarrhea, or you may alternate between the two. Even though the bowel is not damaged, the nerves and muscles of the intestine seem to be oversensitive and overreactive in patients with IBS.

The medical field has yet to determine the cause or causes of IBS. Here's what's known so far: In most patients, it's probably from a "sensitive gut," meaning that people with IBS have increased or exaggerated response to stress or dietary indiscretions. Studies have shown that these patients actually have a higher tolerance of peripheral pain (pain elsewhere in the body) than normal individuals, but their gut is not tolerant to even mild distension. IBS is not a psychological problem; essentially, patients experience gut pain at lower thresholds than the general population. In some patients, IBS seems to develop after a bout of diarrhea from either food poisoning or infection (post-infectious IBS).

Looking at bacterial overgrowth in the small intestine

One cause of IBS may be small intestinal bacterial overgrowth (SIBO). Normally, the small intestine shouldn't have many bacteria, but in IBS bacteria invade the small intestine. Normally, the breakdown of fiber in your gut takes place in the colon, where the gases produced by the breakdown easily escape as flatulence. But in IBS patients, it's postulated that symptoms of gas pains and bloating are because the small intestine's bacteria overgrow, causing the fiber breakdown to occur in the small intestine. There, the gases have no easy escape path.

Bacteria from the colon typically don't invade the small intestine because of peristalsis (waves of contractions in the small intestine that push the bacteria back), and also because the small intestine is more acidic than the colon.

SIBO IBS can be diagnosed with a lactulose breath test, where the patient breathes into a breath collection device. Once diagnosed, IBS can be treated with rifaximin (Xifaxan), a drug that is very minimally absorbed into the bloodstream, acting primarily on the gut, as opposed to other antibiotics that are absorbed into the bloodstream.

After rifaximin, doctors usually give a low dose of erythromycin, which stimulates peristalsis in the small intestine, preventing the bad bacteria from coming back into the small bowel.

Adding probiotics to the IBS mix

There is no specific treatment or "cure" for IBS. Right now, doctors treat the symptoms. Depending on what those are, patients are treated with antispasmodics, antidiarrheals, and/or fiber (including fiber products such as Metamucil, Citrucel, and inulin) and meds that relieve constipation. Tricyclic antidepressants have shown some promise. Dietary adjustments and psychological interventions may help in some (even though it is a true disease of the gut, it's very clear that stress can aggravate the symptoms).

Clinical trials have shown that probiotics can reduce IBS symptoms, especially if the patient has SIBO contributing to IBS. *Bifidobacterium infantis* has been studied extensively and decreases IBS symptoms. A number of other probiotics are effective to a varying degree, but unfortunately with IBS there is so much placebo response that it is difficult to analyze which probiotics truly work and which don't.

In pharmaceutical studies, researchers give a placebo and the drug to the patients in the study. In some cases, patients who receive the placebo report they are better — the *placebo* effect. This effect is particularly high in GI studies (see nearby sidebar for more).

Looking at the placebo effect

When researchers test drugs for safety and effectiveness in controlled studies, participants are typically divided into three groups. One group receives the drug; a second group receives a placebo (or "sugar pill," with no medicinal properties); and the third, or "control," group receives no treatment at all.

The *placebo effect* is the phenomenon of patients (and sometimes even researchers) reporting improvement in symptoms when they haven't received any actual medicine. In *double-blind* studies, where neither the participants nor the researchers know who's receiving the actual drug and who's getting a placebo, the data are less likely to exhibit the placebo effect. However, patients are particularly susceptible, in part because (or so researchers believe) they *want* to believe they feel better.

Right now, there is no proof in medical literature that probiotics after a bout of diarrhea prevent long-term development of IBS. As future research pins down more specific causes of IBS, it is expected that probiotics will play a part in treatment.

Looking at Other Gastrointestinal Disorders

GI problems can be painful and life altering. The good news is that researchers are finding more and more ways to treat GI problems, giving patients options for their healthcare.

Evidence of strides forward is everywhere, even in your grocery store. Just two decades ago, there were very few gluten-free food products on store shelves to help patients diagnosed with celiac disease. Today, entire grocery aisles are dedicated to such products. A similar situation is occurring with probiotics.

Celiac disease

Celiac disease is an autoimmune disorder in which patients develop an allergy to gluten, a protein found in wheat but also in some other grains. Around 1 million Americans have celiac disease. Symptoms include diarrhea, bloating, and weight loss. Diagnosis is made typically by doing blood tests and an upper endoscopy with biopsy of the small intestine, showing changes in the lining.

There is some early evidence that probiotics may help in celiac disease, but research is ongoing. It appears probiotics help in celiac disease by producing chemicals that prevent bacteria from sticking to intestinal cells. This is significant because it appears harmful bacteria stick more tightly to the mucosa in patients with celiac disease.

Peptic ulcers

Ulcers are not uncommon and can occur in the stomach or duodenum. In a majority of patients, ulcers are caused by the *Helicobacter pylori* bacteria. Interestingly, this is the only bacteria found thus far that can survive the acidic media of the stomach.

Ulcers can occur for other reasons, too, such as from stress and non-steroidal anti-inflammatory drugs (NSAIDs, such as Ibuprofen). Probiotics have been found to decrease the number of *H. pylori* bacteria in the stomach. Whether this leads to a decrease in the incidence of ulcers or not is unproven. The treatment for *H. pylori* is antibiotics, and studies have shown that if patients take probiotics along with antibiotics, the chance of eradication of *H. pylori* is higher. (In addition, the chance of getting antibiotic-associated diarrhea and *C. difficile* colitis is also lower.)

Colon cancer

What did Ronald Reagan, Audrey Hepburn, and Pope John Paul II have in common? Colon cancer. This disease is the second leading cause of cancer deaths in the U.S. Around 50,000 people died from colon cancer in 2011. The incidence is almost equal in men and women.

Fortunately, increased screening is causing a reduction in colon cancer incidence over the last 20 years. Most colon cancer starts as colon polyps, which are removed during colonoscopies.

More research needs to be done about how probiotics can help in treating this often deadly disease. Early research indicates that probiotics keep the bad bacteria in check, which appears to help. Bad bacteria can make enzymes that produce carcinogens. Probiotics also may help by stimulating the immune system to destroy abnormal colon cells.

It appears prebiotics play a part in this situation as well, protecting against colon cancer by helping in production of short-chain fatty acids (SCFAs) when they are fermented by the gut bacteria or probiotic. One study compared Africans who eat a high-grain, low-meat diet and African Americans who eat a high-meat diet (a Westernized diet). The high-meat diet eaten by African Americans put them at a higher colon cancer risk compared to the Africans.

Diets high in red meat and animal fat increase the risk of colon cancer. It's possible this is related to gut flora, which alter their metabolic machinery based on what the bacteria is being fed. The byproducts may be toxic and contribute to colon cancer development.

Diets high in prebiotic fibers decrease the risk of colon cancer. Fiber increases the stool bulk and also affects the intestinal transit time. In addition, intestinal bacteria break down the fiber to produce SCFAs. One study found that high butyrate (an SCFA) content in the colon protects against colon cancer. Prebiotics protect against colon cancer by increasing SCFA production.

As in other areas of probiotic research, stay tuned for future developments in this arena.

Lactose intolerance

Lactose is a sugar that occurs naturally in milk. (Sugar in fruit is fructose. Glucose is the sugar produced when you digest carbohydrates, the body's main source of energy. Table sugar is sucrose, which has both glucose and fructose.)

Lactose is a sugar (disaccharide) that contains glucose and galactose, both of which can be absorbed by the small intestinal lining into the bloodstream. The enzyme lactase (also called β-galactosidase) breaks down lactose. Lactose cannot be absorbed.

Lactose intolerance occurs when the level of lactase is low in the small intestine. Lactase activity begins to decrease in childhood or adolescence, and symptoms of lactose intolerance occur. Some diseases of the gut can also cause lactase deficiency.

Thirty to fifty million Americans are lactose intolerant. Fifteen percent of Caucasians are lactose intolerant. The condition is much more prevalent in developing countries in Asia and Africa, where it is estimated that 90 percent of the population is lactose intolerant. Researchers believe the high incidence is attributed to parasitic and/or bacterial infections that are common in these countries.

If you're lactose intolerant and you consume milk or other lactose containing products, symptoms will include bloating, gaseousness, abdominal pain, or cramping and diarrhea. But many people have some lactase and can get by with small quantities of milk. Lactase enzyme supplements are available that help people digest lactose-containing foods easily.

Probiotic research on lactose intolerance shows that *Lactobacillus* and *Bifidobacteria* help reduce symptoms of lactose intolerance. Essentially, probiotics can break down lactose. Even if you're lactose intolerant, you may tolerate lactose-containing foods if you eat them in conjunction with probiotics.

In addition, yogurts containing live active cultures can be a good source of lactase enzymes. Kefir and aged cheeses are also good, as their probiotics also can break down lactose.

Chapter 5

Exploring Allergies and Probiotics

● ●

In This Chapter

▶ Discovering causes of allergies

▶ Understanding asthma and respiratory allergies

▶ Scratching away at eczema

▶ Looking at common food allergies

● ●

*A*bout one in five people globally suffers from some sort of allergic disorder, and the prevalence of allergies continues to rise. For example, the incidence of childhood asthma in the United States increased by 50 percent between 1980 and 2000.

Although environmental factors contribute to allergies, intestinal flora also play a role because, in proper proportion, they help maintain the lining of the digestive system, thus preventing foreign substances from entering the bloodstream.

Several investigators have reported that the makeup of gut flora is different in people who have allergies. In fact, children who live in industrialized countries where allergies are common have different gut flora than children who live in developing countries, where allergies are rare. For example, one study showed that Swedish children have less *Lactobacilli* and *Bifidobacteria* and more *Staphylococcus aureus* (the bacteria that causes staph infections) and *Clostridia* in their bowels than children in Estonia, where allergies aren't as common.

In this chapter, I look at what researchers know about the causes of allergic reactions and explore how the bacteria in your digestive system may help regulate your body's response to allergens. Then I explore several common allergies, including asthma, eczema, and food allergies, and explain how probiotics may help you fight off or ease these allergies.

Understanding the Causes of Allergic Reactions

Allergies are "altered reactions," derived from the Greek words *allos* (meaning different or changed) and *ergos* (meaning work or action).

In medical terms, an allergy is your immune system's exaggerated, usually misguided response to contact with a "foreign" substance. Your body perceives an *allergen* — an allergy-producing substance — as dangerous when it's really not.

Allergies can be mild, moderate, or severe. In some cases, severe allergies can be life threatening, triggering a reaction known as *anaphylaxis*. In anaphylaxis, cells and tissues in your body release chemicals that dilate your blood vessels, which can drop your blood pressure dangerously low. Blood vessels also may leak, causing hives and swelling, particularly in the face and throat. The airways in your lungs constrict, making it harder to breathe (see the section "Looking at Asthma and Respiratory Allergies" later in this chapter).

Anaphylaxis is most commonly caused by

- ✔ Foods, such as peanuts or other kinds of nuts, shellfish, dairy products, and eggs.
- ✔ Stings from bees, wasps, and other insects.
- ✔ Latex.
- ✔ Medications (for example, penicillin).

The hygiene hypothesis

Although no one knows for certain what causes allergic reactions, the *hygiene hypothesis* is the most widely accepted theory in the medical field. The idea is that increasing use of hand sanitizer products means people aren't exposed to microbes as they were decades ago. Childhood exposure to microbes is actually beneficial in the long term because it lessens the likelihood you'll develop allergies. In fact, if you have older siblings, you have a lower chance of developing allergies because you're exposed to more viral infections, which boosts your immune system. There are more allergies in developed countries than in third-world countries — likely because people in less developed areas are exposed to more bacteria and viruses and therefore develop a tolerance for them.

 Anaphylaxis is a medical emergency and requires immediate medical attention. Many people with severe allergies to certain substances carry *epinephrine autoinjectors* (commonly called by the brand name, EpiPen). These are devices that deliver premeasured doses of epinephrine, or adrenaline. Epinephrine quickly constricts blood vessels and relaxes the smooth muscles in the lungs, bringing blood circulation and breathing back to normal. However, even if an epinephrine injection reverses the symptoms of anaphylaxis, the patient should see a doctor to ensure full recovery.

 Most of the time, your body recognizes allergens as harmless and ignores them. But if you're allergic to a particular substance — cat hair, pollen, or mold, for instance — your body snaps to attention, producing an exaggerated response. Fifty million people in the United States have allergies, with nasal allergies, hay fever, asthma, allergic eczema, and hives being the most common.

 Babies born by Caesarian section (C-section) take a long time to achieve bacterial colonization in their digestive system compared to babies born by vaginal delivery, because they aren't exposed to vaginal bacteria (see Chapter 2). Some studies point to increased allergies in children born by C-section.

Looking at Asthma and Respiratory Allergies

When your breathing is normal, you take in air through your nose or mouth (nose breathing is best, by the way, because the hairs in your nose help trap allergens and particles that can cause breathing problems). The air travels down your windpipe to the airways in your lungs, called *bronchial tubes.* Tiny air sacs at the end of the bronchial tubes release oxygen into your bloodstream and collect carbon dioxide, which you release when you exhale.

Bands of muscle wrap around the bronchial tubes. When these muscle bands are relaxed, air moves freely. Several conditions can interfere with normal breathing. In the following sections, I explore some common, chronic respiratory ailments and discuss how probiotics may be related to respiratory health.

Seeing what happens with asthma

In an asthma attack, three main factors make breathing more difficult (see Figure 5-1):

- The muscle bands surrounding the airways tighten, causing the airways to narrow (this reaction is called a *bronchospasm).*
- The airways' lining becomes swollen.
- Cells in the airway lining produce more mucus, which is thicker than normal.

Medicines called *bronchodilators* re-open the airways during an asthma attack and restore normal airflow in and out of the lungs. Asthma usually develops in childhood, and attacks usually are sparked by specific triggers such as allergens. Typically, when the trigger is removed, the asthma attack ends.

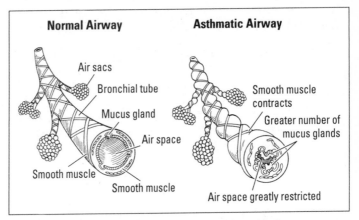

Normal Airway

Asthmatic Airway

Air sacs

Bronchial tube

Mucus gland

Air space

Smooth muscle

Smooth muscle

Smooth muscle contracts

Greater number of mucus glands

Air space greatly restricted

Figure 5-1: Airways are constricted during an asthma attack.

About 16 million American adults and 6 million American children suffer from asthma. According to the American Academy of Allergy, Asthma and Immunology, about half of those people have *allergic asthma*, which means their attacks are triggered by an allergy to, for example, mold spores or pollen. Other triggers for allergic asthma include dust mites, animal dander, and food — especially in children.

Nothing to sneeze at: Hay fever

Hay fever (*allergic rhinitis*) is the most common allergic reaction and can be seasonal or year-round. Symptoms include runny or stuffy nose, sneezing, nasal itching, post-nasal drip, and itchy ears and throat.

Hay fever is an overreaction to harmless particles in the air. Your immune system views pollen or other allergens as dangerous invaders and takes extreme steps to expel them and keep them out. Your bloodstream becomes flooded with chemicals that inflame your sinuses, eyelids, and nasal passages.

People who suffer from hay fever in the spring typically are allergic to tree pollens. Summer sufferers are usually affected by grass and weed pollen, and ragweed is a common hay fever culprit in the fall. Fungus spores can trigger hay fever from late March through November.

Those who have hay fever symptoms year-round are usually allergic to indoor allergens, such as dust mites, animal dander, feathers, and mold.

Hay fever is almost always genetic; most hay fever patients have a parent or sibling who also suffers from allergies. People with asthma or eczema (see the section "Tackling Eczema" later in this chapter) are more likely to develop hay fever. In fact, about one third of those with hay fever also have at least mild allergic asthma.

Using probiotics to promote respiratory health

Researchers have conducted a few studies to see whether probiotics are effective in treating or preventing asthma; so far, most of these studies have focused on treatment options, and the results regarding asthma have been disappointing.

Interestingly, however, one asthma study found that children who received the probiotic *Lactobacillus casei* had fewer episodes of hay fever than a control group. Because asthma and hay fever so often go hand in hand, further research is needed to see whether specific probiotic strains can treat, alleviate, or even prevent asthma.

What do probiotics, which work in your digestive system, have to do with respiratory health? Scientists theorize that the proper balance of good and bad bacteria in your gut help regulate the immune system. Because allergic reactions are essentially overreactions of the immune system, probiotics may play an important role in ensuring that your immune system distinguishes between truly harmful invaders and harmless things like pollen.

Tackling Eczema

Eczema, or *atopic dermatitis,* is the first sign of allergy in the early days of life and is attributed to the immune system's delayed development. This common inflammatory skin disorder in early childhood sometimes continues into adult life. It affects 10–20 percent of infants, but many kids grow out of it by ages 5–15. Forty percent of kids with eczema develop asthma later in childhood.

Probiotics have been successfully used in treatment of eczema. Bacteria studied include *Bifidobacteria* and *Lactobacilli*. According to a study from the Netherlands, daily supplementation with probiotics prevents asthma-like symptoms in children with eczema. In addition, taking prebiotics has been shown to decrease the incidence of eczema in children.

Research studies indicate that if a pregnant woman with eczema takes probiotics during pregnancy, and the newborn is also given probiotics for several months, there is a decreased chance the baby will get eczema.

Chewing on Food Allergies

Food allergies occur when the immune system attacks a food protein. Any food can cause an allergic reaction, but the most common food allergy is sensitivity to peanuts, and sometimes other nuts like pecans and walnuts. Other food allergies include sensitivity to eggs (usually to the proteins in egg whites); cow, goat, and sheep milk or dairy products; and soy, wheat, and shellfish. Mold in foods also can cause allergic reactions — see the nearby sidebar.

Symptoms of food allergies include nausea, vomiting, diarrhea, abdominal pain, hives, and itching. Symptoms can be life threatening when the tongue swells or breathing becomes difficult.

Food allergies aren't the same as food intolerance. For example, many people — especially older people — have trouble digesting milk and some other dairy products because their bodies don't produce enough of the enzyme *lactase*, which breaks down the lactose (sugars) in milk products. Such people are *lactose intolerant* (see Chapter 4), but they aren't allergic to milk.

Breaking out the mold in food

Many people are allergic to mold, and mold spores are everywhere, indoors and out. *Mold* is actually a fungus that digests animal and plant matter, and it's more common in food than you may imagine. In addition, mold develops branches and roots that can penetrate deep inside food, where you can't see it.

If you have an allergic reaction when you eat certain foods, you may actually be allergic to mold in the food rather than the food itself. Common food sources of mold include bread and other foods made with yeast, canned juices, cheese, dried fruits, meats and fish more than 24 hours old, mushrooms, pickled or smoked meats and fish, sauerkraut, sausages (including hot dogs), soy sauce, and vinegar or foods made with vinegar, such as salad dressings. Buttermilk, sour cream, and sour milk also may contain mold.

Mold allergy symptoms are similar to those of other allergies: itchy, watery eyes, stuffy or runny nose, wheezing, and perhaps a rash or hives.

Actual food allergies are relatively rare. About 5 percent of children have some sort of food allergy; in teens and adults, food allergies affect only about 4 percent of the population. As with other allergies, allergies to certain foods involve an overreaction of the immune system to substances that are essentially harmless.

Children are most likely to be allergic to eggs, milk, and peanuts, but they often outgrow these allergies as they get older. In adults, the most common food allergies are

- Peanuts.
- Other tree nuts, such as walnuts, pecans, or cashews.
- Shellfish (crab, crayfish, lobster, and shrimp).
- Milk.
- Eggs.

Most food allergies arise from foods that you eat often. For example, allergy to rice is more common in Japan than in the United States, and codfish allergy is more common in Scandinavia.

Milk and soy allergies are particularly common in infants, but the result typically is *colic* — severe abdominal pain that leads an otherwise healthy baby to cry more than three hours a day, three or more times a week. Babies and young children are believed to be susceptible to milk (and soy) allergies because their immune and digestive systems are immature. Several infant formula manufacturers have begun adding probiotics to their products as aids to digestion and immune system development.

Early research shows that probiotics impact food allergies, but conclusive evidence isn't available yet. Probiotics may be useful in moderating the immune response that occurs during an allergic reaction, decreasing the severity and incidence of allergic disorders. Bacteria studied as being helpful for allergies include *L. plantarum*, *L. rhamnosus*, *L. casei*, and *L. bulgaricus*.

Chapter 6

Getting to the Bottom of Urinary Infections

In This Chapter

▶ Seeing how the urinary system works

▶ Exploring causes and risks for infection

▶ Discovering how probiotics can help with treatment and prevention

*U*rinary tract infections (UTIs) are second only to the common cold in frequency of occurrence. UTIs account for more than 8 million doctor visits in the United States each year. Women are much more prone to these infections than men, though no one is quite sure why. Most urinary tract infections are simple and easy to treat, but the treatment — a course of antibiotics — can wreak havoc with the microbial balance in your digestive system.

In this chapter, I show you how the urinary system works and how infections can arise. I provide some tips on preventing infections and look at how and why probiotics can help keep you out of the doctor's office — at least for a urinary tract infection.

Understanding Your Urinary System

Although men and women have different physiology, the basic structure of their urinary systems is the same. This system consists of the kidneys, ureters (the tubes that carry urine from the kidneys to the bladder), the bladder, and the urethra, which allows you to eliminate urine from your body. Figure 6-1 shows the basics of the human urinary system.

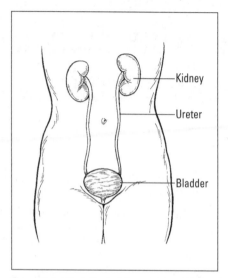

Figure 6-1: Front view of the urinary system.

The kidneys filter a substance called *urea,* as well as excess water and other waste, from your blood. Muscles in the ureter walls continually contract and expand to move urine from the kidneys to the bladder; when these muscles don't work properly, urine can back up in the kidneys and cause an infection.

Aging, injury, and illness can cause problems in the urinary system. For example, as you get older, the muscles in your bladder may lose strength, so they don't tighten enough to empty your bladder completely — which can cause bladder infections. Anything that obstructs the flow of urine can cause a UTI. An enlarged prostate, a situation common in men as they age, can also cause a UTI.

Illness or injury also can affect the kidneys and prevent them from thoroughly filtering the blood — or can block the flow of urine into the bladder.

In the following sections, I look at common causes and risk factors for urinary tract infections and how they're treated.

Looking at infections

UTIs can occur anywhere in the urinary system, and they are the second most common type of infection.

Urine normally is *sterile*, meaning it's free of bacteria, viruses, and fungi. To help ward off infections, the ureters and bladder prevent urine from backing up to the kidneys, and the flow of urine through the urethra helps wash away any bacteria. In men, the prostate gland also secretes substances that inhibit bacterial growth, and in both sexes, other immune functions help keep the urinary system healthy.

Infections often occur when bacteria from the digestive tract — especially *E. coli*, which normally lives in the colon (see Chapter 2) — cling to the opening of the urethra and multiply. Other bacteria, including *Chlamydia* and *Mycoplasma,* can also cause UTIs. However, unlike *E. coli, Chlamydia* and *Mycoplasma* can be sexually transmitted, which means both partners should be treated.

Women tend to get UTIs more often than men. In fact, women have a 50 percent chance of developing a UTI in their lifetime, and 20 percent have recurring UTIs. No one knows for sure why women are so susceptible to UTIs. One theory is that the female urethra is short, so bacteria don't have to travel as far to the bladder. The fact that the urethra opening is so close to the vagina and anus also may play a role. In addition, this anatomic difference has hormonal effects, and behavioral patterns in women may also contribute to the increased risk.

UTIs are less common in males, especially boys and young men. However, when men do get a UTI, it can be more serious.

Risk factors for UTIs include the following:

- ✔ **Abnormalities in the urinary tract.** Kidney stones and other abnormalities can interfere with the flow of urine, setting the stage for an infection. In men, an enlarged prostate also can slow urine flow.

- ✔ **Catheters.** Catheters are tubes placed in the urethra and bladder — used when a patient can't empty the bladder normally, as sometimes happens with spinal cord injuries, or when the patient is unconscious or critically ill. If not properly sanitized, bacteria on the catheter can cause a UTI.

- ✔ **Diabetes and immune disorders.** When your immune system is compromised, it can't fight off foreign invaders as efficiently. People with diabetes often have a lower immune response than healthy people.

- ✔ **Diaphragm use.** Several studies have linked UTIs to the use of a diaphragm for birth control. In addition, researchers recently found that women whose partners use condoms with spermicidal foam for contraception tend to have *E. coli* growth in the vagina — another risk factor for both UTIs and vaginal infections (see Chapter 7).

- ✔ **Pregnancy.** Pregnant women seem to be more susceptible to UTIs, and these infections can be more serious because they're more likely to travel to the kidneys in pregnant women.

UTI symptoms may include frequent urination, painful urination, an urgent feeling of having to go to the bathroom, fever, chills, and/or cloudy urine. If you have pain in the area below the ribs, on your side, it may mean the UTI has gone to your kidneys (called pyelonephritis). A UTI involving the urethra is called urethritis, and one involving the bladder is cystitis.

Treating UTIs

Because most UTIs are caused by bacterial infections, treatment consists of (can you guess?) antibiotics. Both the specific antibiotic and the length of treatment depend on the patient's history and which bacteria are causing the infection.

Antibiotics don't distinguish between beneficial and harmful bacteria; they kill off both kinds. So many doctors now prescribe probiotic supplements along with antibiotics to help repopulate the good bacteria in your digestive tract (see Chapter 2).

Simple UTIs — that is, infections that aren't complicated by an obstruction or other problem — often can be cured in a day or two with antibiotics. However, many doctors prescribe antibiotics for between 7 and 14 days to ensure the infection is wiped out.

In some cases — and especially for women who have three or more UTIs per year — doctors prescribe low-dose antibiotics for six months or longer. If your doctor recommends this

course of treatment for you, probiotic supplen
more important.

You can take steps to help prevent UTIs:

- ✔ Drink lots of water every day.

- ✔ Urinate when you feel the urge; remember, urinating helps wash bacteria from the urethra.

- ✔ Wipe from front to back; this technique helps prevent bacteria around the anus from migrating to the vagina or urethra.

- ✔ Clean your genital area before intercourse (and your doctor may advise you to take a single antibiotic dose after intercourse, because intercourse is a risk factor for UTIs).

- ✔ Take showers instead of baths (bacteria from the anus can migrate in bath water).

- ✔ Don't use douches or feminine washes; these products upset the bacterial balance in your vagina (see Chapter 7) and can promote the growth of harmful bacteria.

Some doctors suggest drinking cranberry juice.

Bringing Probiotics to the Fight

Research shows that women who consume fermented milk products containing probiotics (such as kefir) have a lower incidence of UTIs. A recent U.S. study showed that recurrent UTIs were markedly reduced in women who used vaginal suppositories containing probiotics.

Whenever you take antibiotics for a UTI or other bacterial infection, the drugs kill off friendly bacteria in your gut (see Chapter 2). Taking probiotics along with antibiotics can reduce your chances of having antibiotic-related diarrhea. But, just as important, probiotics can help neutralize the bad effects of antibiotics.

As I mentioned earlier, research is uncovering some evidence that probiotic intake can help prevent UTIs in the first place — possibly because when you have enough good bacteria in your system, the bad bacteria don't have a chance to proliferate. You can add probiotics to your daily routine by choosing probiotics-rich foods (see Chapter 11 and the recipes in Chapter 12), or by taking probiotic supplements.

Chapter 7

Using Probiotics in Women's Health

*R*esearch on probiotics has yielded some promising results for women's health. Although probiotics are generally safe — and often beneficial — for everyone, they can be particularly effective in preventing or treating many symptoms and ailments unique to women.

In this chapter, you discover how probiotics can alleviate some of the unpleasant side effects of pregnancy and convey benefits to both the developing fetus and infants. In addition, studies have demonstrated that probiotics can help prevent or treat common "female problems," such as certain vaginal infections and urinary tract infections.

Probiotics and Pregnancy

Pregnancy generates a host of changes in a woman's body, and some of the side effects of those changes can be quite unpleasant. However, researchers are providing increasing evidence that probiotics can help alleviate some of the most common digestive and other issues with pregnancy. Some studies also indicate that developing fetuses benefit when pregnant women increase their probiotic intake. And probiotics also may help protect infants against colic, eczema, and other problems.

Studies show that consuming probiotics during pregnancy offers several advantages for mom and baby. Mom

- ✔ Is 18 percent less likely to deliver a preterm baby.
- ✔ Loses baby weight faster after delivery.
- ✔ Is less likely to develop *central obesity* (belly fat).
- ✔ Has a 20 percent lower chance of developing *gestational diabetes* (the presence of high blood sugar during pregnancy that increases the risk of subsequent development of diabetes after pregnancy).

The baby

- ✔ Has a lower risk of developing a serious condition called *necrotizing enterocolitis*, or the death of intestinal tissue.
- ✔ Is 50 percent less likely to get eczema.
- ✔ Is less likely to develop asthma.
- ✔ Has a decreased chance of developing childhood obesity and diabetes.

Rebalancing mom's digestive system

Pregnancy often wreaks havoc with a woman's digestive system. Heartburn, constipation, diarrhea, nausea, and vomiting are common issues, especially during the first trimester.

Hormonal changes, fatigue, and stress upset the balance of good and bad bacteria in the gut (see Chapter 2), so your digestive system doesn't work as efficiently. Probiotics — consumed through diet or supplements, or both — help restore the proper bacterial balance and digestive function.

Always consult with your physician before adding any supplements, including probiotics, to your diet. Your doctor may have recommendations for specific probiotics to take.

Pregnant women also often suffer from urinary tract infections (see Chapter 6), yeast infections (covered later in this chapter), and skin inflammation — all of which can be prevented or eased by taking probiotics.

Gaining weight after birth

Many women retain "belly fat" after giving birth, and excess belly fat is associated with several serious health issues, including cardiovascular disease.

One study in Finland followed 256 women from the first trimester of their pregnancies to a year after they gave birth. The women were split into three groups: one group received dietary counseling and probiotic supplements, the second group received counseling and a placebo, and the third group received the placebo with no counseling.

A year after giving birth, the women who received the probiotics had the lowest percentage of body fat and the lowest incidence of belly fat. Only 25 percent of the probiotics group had *central obesity* — defined as a body mass index of 30 or higher and a waist measurement of 31.5 inches or more. But 43 percent of the women who got dietary counseling and a placebo had central obesity a year after giving birth, as did 40 percent of the women who received the placebo and no dietary advice.

 Probiotics' role in weight management isn't clear yet, but researchers have found that the makeup of gut flora differs between lean and obese people. See Chapter 9 for more on probiotics and weight management.

Giving baby's health a boost

Research indicates that developing fetuses benefit when mom takes probiotics during pregnancy. Probiotics during pregnancy help promote a stronger immune system at birth. In addition, probiotics reduce the risk of mom developing gestational diabetes, which is one of the most causes of large babies. Babies who are big at birth (generally weighing more than 8 pounds, 13 ounces, or who are in the 85th or higher percentile of height and weight measurements) are at higher risk for becoming overweight later in life. (See Chapter 8 for more on childhood obesity and probiotics.)

Even though breast feeding is the best form of feeding, formulas are indispensable in situations when mothers cannot feed their children. Studies have shown that daily feeding with a prebiotic-enriched baby formula produced gut bacteria that "closely resembled" those of breast-fed infants. Today more and more formulas now include probiotics, prebiotics, and *synbiotics* (combinations of prebiotics and probiotics).

Probiotics also may help alleviate the symptoms of *colic* — severe abdominal pain that leads an otherwise healthy baby to cry more than three hours a day, three or more times a week. No one really knows what causes colic, but recent research indicates that bacterial imbalance in the gut may lead to inflammation. One study found that colicky babies had both inflammation and traces of bacteria that may have caused it, whereas babies without colic had no inflammation and more varieties of good bacteria in their gut. Other studies have shown that the probiotic *Lactobacillus reuteri* decreased crying in colicky babies to less than an hour a day, compared with two and a half hours of crying for colicky babies who were given medication to reduce gas.

 L. reuteri is found in breast milk, and Canadian researchers reported that this good bacterium decreases the force of muscle contractions in the gut. This research may help explain why colicky babies cry less when treated with this probiotic: they don't experience as much painful cramping.

Using Probiotics in Urogenital Infections

More than 75 percent of women have less-than-optimal vaginal health, and a third of them test positive for *bacterial vaginosis,* an infection caused by an imbalance in vaginal bacteria. Normally, *Lactobacillus* is the predominant bacteria in the vagina, and it's considered protective in several ways. *Lactobacilli* adhere to the vaginal epithelial cells, preventing bad bacteria from adhering, and also produce chemicals such as lactic acid and hydrogen peroxide, which inhibit other bad bacteria when there is an imbalance. Bacterial imbalances increase risks for urinary tract infections (UTIs), bacterial vaginosis, yeast infections, sexually transmitted diseases (STDs), and pre-term labor.

When they have a vaginal problem, many women self-medicate using over-the-counter yeast infection treatments.

Unfortunately, these treatments may not be effective and can even be counterproductive, actually *increasing* the colonization of harmful bacteria (see Chapter 1).

Research has found that probiotics help in treating or preventing many urogenital infections. Probiotic vaginal suppositories are frequently used outside the United States and seem to work better than oral probiotics. A Swedish company, Ellen AB, manufactures a patented probiotic tampon and claims it strengthens women's defenses against infection.

In the following sections, I look at three common urogenital problems: bacterial vaginosis, yeast infections, and urinary tract infections.

Battling bacterial vaginosis

Bacterial vaginosis (BV) is the most common cause of vaginal infections — not to be confused with a yeast infection. Symptoms include an off-white vaginal discharge, often accompanied by an unpleasant smell. Treating BV with antibiotics helps only 40 percent of women, but results are better when probiotics are added to the treatment.

Cigarette smoking, use of IUDs, frequent douches, and multiple sex partners increase the incidence of BV. Use of spermicides can kill friendly *Lactobacilli* and increase incidence of BV.

Multiple research reports show the benefits of using *L. acidophilus* to treat BV; in many studies, the probiotic was administered via vaginal suppositories. A smaller number of studies found that eating yogurt enriched with *L. acidophilus* may be beneficial, but results weren't definitive.

There is evidence that continuous use of probiotics by women who have had BV decreases future incidence of BV. It's also wise for women who've had a history of BV or yeast infections to take probiotics whenever they take antibiotics.

Tamping down yeast infections

Most women — about 3 in 4 — will have a yeast infection at least once in their lives. These fungal infections are typically caused by *Candida albicans*. Symptoms of a yeast infection include a whitish discharge, vaginal itching, and soreness.

Women who have diabetes are particularly susceptible to yeast infections. In one small study, women who ate six ounces of frozen, artificially sweetened, live-culture yogurt a day reported fewer yeast infections and were found to have normal vaginal pH balances (a measure of how acidic something is). Women who ate frozen yogurt without live cultures had high vaginal pH levels at the beginning and end of the study.

Yeast infections often occur after antibiotic treatment, but can also occur after steroid use, while using birth control pills, and with frequent douching. Stress is also a common cause of yeast infections. Treatment typically consists of using an anti-fungal medication such as miconazole (sold under the brand names Aloe Vesta, Baza, and Cruex Prescription Strength) or clotrimazole (Lotrimin and Gyne-Lotrimin, Desenex, and so on) as a topical cream or orally.

L. acidophilus, *L. rhamnosus*, and *L. fermentum* have been shown to prevent and treat yeast infections. Many doctors are beginning to recommend that patients take a probiotic along with antibiotic prescriptions, particularly women who have a history of yeast infections.

Squelching urinary tract infections

Urinary tract infections (UTIs) are caused by a bacterial infection anywhere in the urinary tract. Symptoms include frequent need to urinate, pain during urination, and sometimes cloudy urine. Women are more prone to UTIs than men, with 50 percent developing the infection during their lifetime. Half of those women will have recurrent problems. Having frequent intercourse, being female, and using catheters all increase the risk of UTIs.

The most common organism causing UTIs is the *E. coli* bacterium. The usual treatment is a short round of antibiotics. Research shows that women who consume fermented milk products containing probiotics (such as yogurt and kefir) have a lower incidence of UTIs. A recent U.S. study showed that recurrent UTIs were markedly reduced in women who used vaginal suppositories containing probiotics. For detailed information about UTIs and probiotics, see Chapter 6.

Chapter 8

Understanding Children's Health and Probiotics

. . . .

In This Chapter

▶ Giving infants good bacteria for healthy immune system

▶ Treating acute diarrhea in children

▶ Preventing and treating childhood asthma

▶ Offering hope for autism

▶ Tackling the obesity epidemic

. . . .

*C*hildren's immune systems aren't fully developed. Kids are continuously challenged by environmental factors such as infections (both bacterial and viral) at daycare centers and schools, allergens and irritants in foods, chemical toxins, and antibiotic use. All these factors make probiotics even more important for children than they are for adults. Probiotics not only improve their digestive functions but also help support their weaker immune functions. Probiotics may even decrease allergy sensitivity in children.

Several studies indicate that giving probiotics to children at an early age reduces the severity and duration of a variety of diseases. For example, some studies reported that colds and flus decreased by 50 percent, and diarrhea from viral infections also decreased after using probiotics.

Autism and childhood obesity are of special interest in the study of how probiotics may help children. Although the research is far from complete, scientists are looking at how these conditions may be related to bacteria in the body. In this chapter, I explore the various ways probiotics may help improve your child's health from infancy into adulthood.

Looking at Infants' Special Needs

Babies are fragile in many ways, and their immune systems are no exception. For the first six months, infants rely on their mother's antibodies — passed on through breast milk — to help them build up their immune systems. One reason that breast milk is preferable to powdered formula is that, even though most of today's formulas contain special proteins and nutrients designed for a baby's delicate digestive system, manufacturers haven't yet found a reliable way to duplicate the antibodies present in breast milk.

Some research suggests that breast-fed babies are less likely than formula-fed babies to develop certain infections — especially respiratory and ear infections, as well as diarrhea — during their first year.

One of the most critical antibodies infants get from breast milk is *Immunoglobulin A*, or IgA, which protects the body surfaces that are often exposed to foreign — and potentially harmful — organisms from outside the body. IgA antibodies are prevalent in the nose and airways, the digestive tract, ears, eyes, saliva, and tears. Breast-fed babies benefit by receiving their mothers' IgA to help them fend off disease and infection.

Breast milk contains four other types of immunoglobulin:

- ✔ **IgD:** IgD antibodies are found in small quantities in the lining of the abdominal and chest cavities, and in smaller quantities in the bloodstream. Researchers believe IgD plays a role in allergic reactions to things like milk, medications, and poisons.

- ✔ **IgE:** IgE antibodies are in the lungs, skin, and mucous membranes. They induce reactions to allergens such as pollen, fungus, and mold spores, and animal dander. People with hay fever or other allergies often have high levels of IgE antibodies (see Chapter 5).

- ✔ **IgG:** IgG antibodies are the most common, comprising between 75 and 80 percent of all antibodies in your system. They're in all body fluids and are a critical force in fighting off both bacterial and viral infections. Because they're so small, they're the only antibodies that can pass through the placenta, helping the developing fetus fight off infection in the womb.

✓ **IgM:** IgM antibodies are the largest; they reside in the bloodstream and lymph fluids. When your body detects an infection, it begins producing IgM antibodies as a first response. IgM antibodies also trigger other cells in the immune system to produce compounds to help fight off foreign invaders.

Breast milk also contains prebiotic *oligosaccharides* — sugar molecules that provide food for probiotic bacteria. These molecules also prevent harmful bacteria from multiplying; they bind with bad bacteria, forming a compound that the baby excretes as waste. Oligosaccharides also have been shown to lower the incidence of eczema among infants, especially when taken during the first six months (see Chapter 5 for more information on probiotics and eczema).

Healthy babies start producing their own antibodies at between two and three months. However, because infants initially produce antibodies at a slow pace, they go through a period where the number of antibodies in their system is low. By the time a healthy baby is six months old, its body begins producing antibodies at a normal rate.

According to a study published in the *American Journal of Clinical Nutrition*, infants who took probiotic-supplemented formula had a lower rate of colic and needed fewer antibiotics.

Although breastfeeding is still considered the gold standard, infant formula has long been considered a "good enough" substitute. In recent years, formula manufacturers in the United States have begun adding probiotics and prebiotic nutrients to their formulas. Check out Gerber's Good Start Protect (www. gerber.com) and Enfamil Premium (www.enfamil.com).

Battling Acute Pediatric Diarrhea

Diarrhea is common in children, but it also can be extremely serious because children dehydrate more quickly than adults. In the United States, 16.5 million children under the age of 5 have one bout of diarrhea a year, and about 10 percent of those children require hospitalization. Outside the U.S., the statistics are worse: More than 3 million children die of acute infectious diarrhea every year, mainly in developing countries.

Several studies indicate that giving children probiotic supplements at the onset of diarrhea can shorten the duration of the illness by as much as a day; hospital stays also are shorter when probiotics are administered. In addition, when probiotics are given in conjunction with antibiotics, children are less susceptible to subsequent infection because the probiotics replace the good bacteria that the antibiotics wipe out (see Chapter 4 for more on antibiotics' effects on gut flora). Evidence also suggests that probiotics help keep inflammation under control.

So far, the probiotic *Lactobacillus rhamnosus GG* has shown the most consistent benefits in treating acute pediatric diarrhea. However, researchers continue to examine other probiotic species and strains to see how effective they may be.

Keeping Children Well

Childhood exposure to microbes is beneficial in the long term because it lessens the likelihood you'll develop allergies. In fact, if you have older siblings, you have a lower chance of developing allergies because you're exposed to more viral infections, which boosts your immune system. There are more allergies in developed countries than in developing countries — likely because people in less developed areas are exposed to more bacteria and viruses and therefore develop a tolerance.

Probiotics and prebiotics can help support children's immune systems, too. Research into which probiotic species and strains (see Chapter 3) are best for children is not advanced. However, early evidence suggests that the following probiotics are beneficial for both infants and children:

- *Bifidobacterium bifidum*
- *Bifidobacterium lactis*
- *Lactobacillus acidophilus*
- *Lactobacillus reuteri*
- *Lactobacillus rhamnosus GG* (marketed as Culturelle Probiotic for Kids)
- *Saccharomyces boulardii* (probiotic yeast)

Based on the hygiene hypothesis (see Chapter 5), kids who aren't exposed to enough microorganisms to stimulate their immune system could benefit from probiotics. So doesn't it make sense for every kid born in the United States to be on probiotics — or at least eat probiotic-rich foods? (Turn to Chapter 11 to find which foods are packed with prebiotics and probiotics; then see Chapter 12 for great probiotic recipes.)

Aside from promoting general good health, probiotics may have a role to play in helping with three critical childhood health issues: asthma, autism, and obesity. Although the research is far from complete, scientists are looking at how these conditions may be related to bacteria in the body. I take a closer look in the following sections.

Breathing easy: Asthma and probiotics

Asthma is a common chronic childhood disease; in fact, it's one of the most common reasons that kids miss school. *Asthma* is inflammation of the bronchial tubes in the lungs, which obstructs the airway and causes coughing, wheezing, and a feeling of tightness in the chest.

Research indicates that asthma, like eczema, is linked to an abnormal immune response. "Leaky gut" syndrome (see Chapter 4) allows allergens to pass through the intestinal wall into the bloodstream and is associated with allergies. Probiotics can help because they promote the integrity of the intestinal walls and help regulate immune system responses.

In addition to treating existing asthma, probiotics also show promise for asthma prevention. In one study, pregnant women who had at least one first-degree relative or partner with eczema, allergies, or asthma were given the probiotic *Lactobacillus rhamnosus GG* until six months after giving birth. Their babies had only half the incidence of infant eczema compared with the infants of women who took a placebo. Because infant eczema is linked to childhood asthma, this study seems promising for preventing asthma.

Autism and probiotics

Autism Spectrum Disorders is a group of neural development disorders characterized by impaired social interactions and communication, emotional outbursts, and restrictive and repetitive behaviors. Signs of autism usually develop gradually, and parents begin noticing it in the first two years of a child's life. Occasionally, children may show normal development and then regress. An estimated 500,000 people in the United States suffer from some degree of autism.

Autism has a strong genetic connection, but early research indicates that it may be exacerbated by environmental factors like toxins, antibiotics, bacteria, viruses, and nutritional deficiencies. Although research on the use of probiotics and autism is still in its infancy, there is some indication that gut bacteria is different in individuals exhibiting autism symptoms, and interest is growing in exploring the role of gut pathology may play in this disorder.

One study indicated a link between autism and certain gut bacteria. And in another study, autistic children who took a probiotic supplement showed such marked improvement that their parents withdrew their children from the study rather than take them off the probiotics as required by the rigors of a blind clinical trial. Unfortunately, the drop-out rate meant the study had to be scrapped, and thus there's no scientifically valid claim of probiotics' effectiveness in treating the symptoms of autism. However, the not-so-blind study does give hope to millions of parents of autistic children.

Childhood obesity

Childhood obesity is on the rise; one in three kids in the United States is obese. Babies who are big at birth (generally weighing more than 8 pounds, 13 ounces, or in the 85th or higher percentile of height-and-weight measurements) are at higher risk for becoming overweight later in life. Studies have found that women who take probiotics during pregnancy (see Chapter 7) have a decreased risk of developing gestational diabetes, one of the most common causes of large babies.

Breast-fed babies are at a lower risk for later obesity than non-breast fed babies. Scientists also know that *Bifidobacteria* are prevalent in the guts of breast-fed babies. As in adults, it appears that lean children have higher levels of *Bifidobacteria*.

Chapter 9

Applying Probiotics to Other Health Issues

Twenty years ago, the concept of probiotics was little understood. Today, as research accumulates and the role of probiotics is defined, U.S. doctors are beginning to use probiotics and prebiotics to treat a variety of diseases.

The next step in probiotic and prebiotic research is to determine how they can be used to prevent disease. As the critical role of gut flora in optimal health becomes more evident, it's clear that there's tremendous potential in adding good bacteria to your diet.

In this chapter, you discover what research is showing about how probiotics can help prevent or treat a wide range of diseases and conditions — from certain types of cancer to heart, kidney, and liver disease — as well as how probiotics may help promote weight management.

Exploring Cancer Prevention

Few words in the medical world are more ominous than *cancer*. Tremendous advances in the past few decades have changed the way cancers are treated, upping the success rates for some cancers. Research also is delving into what you can do to prevent cancer, aside from the obvious things like avoiding cigarettes that can lead to lung cancer and high-fat diets that can lead to colon cancer.

That research has identified things you can do to increase the odds that you won't get particular kinds of cancer. A high-fiber diet helps protect against colon cancer, for example.

In the following sections, I discuss the current understanding of how cancer works and why it's so tough to beat, as well as explore intriguing research indicating that probiotics may help prevent certain types of cancer.

Understanding current cancer theory

"Cancer" is actually a collection of about 100 diseases that share some characteristics but differ in ways that make treatment challenging. In simple terms, *cancer* occurs when normal cells become abnormal as a result of genetic changes. Sometimes these genetic changes are inherited, but most often they occur because of environmental factors: diet, behaviors such as smoking, or exposure to harsh chemicals, pollutants, and even certain viruses.

Unlike normal cells, cancer cells

- Don't stop growing when they should.
- Don't die when they should.
- Divide more often and more rapidly than they should.
- Can migrate to other parts of the body and lie dormant for lengthy periods.

Cancer treatment typically consists of surgery, radiation, or chemotherapy — or some combination of these options. The problem with current treatments is that they all damage or destroy healthy, normal cells in addition to the cancer cells. Researchers are looking for ways to better target just cancer cells; meanwhile, other researchers are trying to determine ways you can prevent cancer cells from forming in the first place.

Seeing how probiotics may prevent cancer

Initial studies of the effects of probiotics on cancer appear promising. In one series of experiments, for example, two groups of rats were fed cancer-causing agents, but the rats in Group I were given probiotics. Group I rats didn't develop tumors, whereas the second group did.

The probiotic anti-cancer effect may be related to increased production of short-chain fatty acids (SCFA). One SCFA, *butyrate*, inhibits the growth of cancer cells and stimulates activity of an enzyme that acts as a detoxification system for potentially harmful compounds.

Combating colon cancer

Colon cancer is the second-leading cause of cancer deaths. Animal and *in vitro* (meaning in a culture dish in a lab) studies have shown that probiotics may lower colon cancer risk by reducing the incidence and number of tumors.

Preliminary data suggests that *Lactobacilli* and *Bifidobacteria* prevent mutation in genes, decreasing colon cancer incidence. Animals that received *Lactobacillus rhamnosus GG* showed a reduction in the activity of bacterial enzymes that play a role in causing cancer.

The data from human trials is circumstantial, and more studies are required to determine whether probiotics reduce the chance of developing colon cancer or slow its progression. However, three studies have shown positive indications for using probiotics and prebiotics to prevent and treat colon cancer.

A study published in the *American Journal of Clinical Nutrition* found that foods fortified with probiotics and prebiotics reduced certain markers of colon cancer in patients who already had colon cancer. This study provides the most direct evidence to date that the combination of probiotics and prebiotics benefits patients with colon cancer.

Studies in humans often take several years to complete. One quick way to get an assessment of a treatment's effectiveness is to use *biomarkers* — characteristics of cells or molecules that can be objectively measured — to determine levels of *toxic metabolites,* which are potentially harmful substances formed as the result of normal body functions. A Belgian study that used this method reported that consuming either a probiotic (*Lactobacillus* or *Bifidobacterium*) or a prebiotic (oligofructose or inulin) resulted in reduced levels of specific toxic metabolites.

Finally, in a European study of human patients, one group took a mixture of probiotics and prebiotics for eight weeks. They had less DNA damage and a lower rate of cell proliferation in their colon tissue samples than a control group, which didn't take probiotics or prebiotics. In addition, stool samples from the probiotics group had certain characteristics that indicated reduced cancer risk.

Considering bladder cancer

Bladder cancer is common and typically has a high recurrence rate. One clinical study found that patients with bladder cancer who took probiotics (*Lactobacillus casei*) had longer remission periods, in which the cancer didn't reappear.

A Japanese study also found that cancer patients who received probiotics took longer to develop the cancer, and that the cancers were not as severe when they recurred in probiotic-treated patients.

Treating cervical cancer

Treatment for cervical cancer consists of surgery in the early stages and chemotherapy and radiotherapy in the advanced stages.

One study of 228 women with advanced cervical cancer found that those who received probiotics had a higher four-year survival rate — 69 percent versus 46 percent for women who didn't receive probiotics.

Another study found that when probiotics were given before and during radiation for cervical cancer, patients had less radiation-related diarrhea. Nine percent of the probiotic group needed antidiarrhea medication, whereas 32 percent of the non-probiotic group needed antidiarrheals.

Slowing down lung cancer

Initial research shows that probiotics don't reduce the incidence of lung cancer, but may slow its growth. Cancer cell growth in lung cancer patients who received vitamin K2 was slower than in patients who didn't take the vitamin.

Probiotics may play a role here because they convert vitamin K1, which is common in vegetables, to vitamin K2 in the colon (which may reduce the risk of colon cancer).

Treating Heart Disease

Fifty percent of all deaths in United States are caused by heart disease and strokes. The most common factors contributing to these illnesses are high cholesterol, smoking, high blood pressure, and diabetes.

The following sections discuss how probiotics may help alleviate these contributing factors.

Lowering blood pressure

Fifty million Americans have high blood pressure, often called "the silent killer" because many people have no symptoms. Blood pressure is measured in two ways:

- ✔ *Systolic* is the pressure when your heart beats while it's pumping blood
- ✔ *Diastolic* is the pressure of blood pushing against the walls of your arteries between heartbeats.

Normal blood pressure is 120/80 (systolic/diastolic) or lower.

High blood pressure can damage your arteries and other blood vessels, as well as your heart, kidneys, and other organs.

Milk proteins have properties that help fight high blood pressure. Probiotic enzymes break down milk proteins into useable components. Animal studies show that the probiotic *Lactobacilli* can reduce blood pressure.

Keeping cholesterol in balance

Cholesterol has a good component (HDL) and a bad component (LDL). The higher the LDL levels, the higher the risk of heart disease. HDL, on the other hand, protects against heart disease.

Probiotics can break down cholesterol and use it in their metabolic processes, which decrease your cholesterol levels. Fermented milk and *L. acidophilus* have been shown to increase HDL and lower LDL, decreasing the chance of heart disease, and other studies have shown that *L. acidophilus and L. lactis* decrease cholesterol.

Probiotics also may decrease cholesterol by lowering the synthesis of cholesterol by the liver. Your liver uses cholesterol to make bile acids. Bile is stored in the liver and, when needed, pumped into the small bowel, where 95 percent of the bile is reabsorbed and makes its way back to the liver.

Probiotics make an enzyme that breaks down the bile salts that can't be reabsorbed. The liver then reaches out into the blood to get new cholesterol, which lowers the amount of cholesterol in the blood. All *Bifidobacteria* species, *Lactobacillus acidophilus,* and some other *Lactobacilli* have this capability.

 Adding prebiotics to probiotics helps probiotics flourish (see Chapter 1), but prebiotics — because they're fiber — also directly work to decrease cholesterol.

Using Probiotics in Fighting Kidney and Liver Disease

The liver and kidneys get toxins out of your system and process nutrients from the foods you eat. Any interruption of the functioning of these two organs, whether through disease or more short-term illnesses, can cause serious health problems.

Breaking down kidney stones

About 1 in 20 Americans suffer from kidney stones at some point in their lives. Men tend to have more kidney stones than women, and stones tend to recur; in fact, for some, kidney stones are a lifelong problem. Sometimes kidney stones present no symptoms; other times, they cause severe pain and blood in the urine. In some cases, kidney stones can lead to kidney failure.

The most common type of stone (more than 80 percent of cases) is composed of *calcium oxalate,* a chemical compound that forms needle-shaped crystals. Your gut bacteria — primarily *Oxalobacter formigenes*, but also *B. lactis, L. acidophilus,* and *B. infantis* — normally break down oxalate. However, if you don't have these gut bacteria in adequate amounts, then your gut absorbs the oxalate and the burden of excreting it falls on the kidneys. When your kidneys can't excrete oxalate fast enough, you can develop kidney stones.

Probiotics help patients with kidney stones by breaking down the oxalate so it doesn't go to the kidney in the first place. A University of Boston study found that people who have a lot of *Oxalobacter formigenes* in their systems are 70 percent less likely to develop kidney stones.

In animal studies, oral probiotics improve kidney function by decreasing both *blood urea nitrogen* and *serum creatinine* levels. Probiotics have been used in cats and dogs for kidney failure for a long time.

Early evidence suggests that probiotics can postpone dialysis for people with kidney failure. But you'll have to stay tuned as more research is done on that issue.

Improving liver function

Your liver processes alcohol, drugs (including over-the-counter medications like ibuprofen), and toxins. Several prescription drugs are particularly harmful to the liver and can result in fatty deposits in the liver. Being overweight or obese also can generate fatty deposits in the liver, which can lead to inflammation, scarring, and even liver failure.

People who consume a lot of alcohol (more than two drinks per day for men, and more than one drink a day for women) are at particularly high risk for developing liver disease. But even nondrinkers can get liver disease, because the liver receives virtually all the blood flow from the digestive tract.

So any toxins that you take in through food, drink, or drugs go through the liver.

Preliminary evidence indicates that probiotics reduce the absorption of *aflatoxin,* which is strongly linked to liver cancer, from the intestine. Probiotics may have a role to play in preventing liver cancer in people with *cirrhosis* (a chronic disease in which the liver is inflamed and scarred, usually from alcohol abuse or liver disease caused by toxins or viruses), who are at high risk for developing liver cancer.

End-stage liver disease, caused by various issues, can cause *hepatic encephalopathy,* which means toxins like ammonia aren't pushed out by the liver and thus affect the patient's nervous system. Cirrhosis patients have substantially altered gut flora, with overgrowth of disease-causing *E. coli* and *Staphylococcus* bacteria. In one study, probiotics increased the *Lactobacilli* species in the gut, and this increase was associated with decreased blood ammonia levels and decreased encephalopathy.

As the studies pile up, the role of probiotics in promoting healthy liver function is promising. But more human trials are needed in this arena.

Promoting Immune Function

About 90 percent of your immune system is located in your digestive tract (see Chapter 1). Normally, your immune system recognizes and gets rid of harmful bacteria, viruses, and toxins, while leaving the "good" or harmless stuff alone.

In *autoimmune* diseases, the immune system attacks healthy cells and organisms. And, at least in some autoimmune diseases, an imbalance between good and bad gut flora (see Chapter 1) may be at least partially to blame.

Developed countries have a higher incidence of some autoimmune conditions such as Type 1 diabetes (often called *juvenile diabetes*). A low intake of prebiotic fiber adversely affects the intestinal microbiota, which leads to less production of elements that regulate the immune system, such as short-chain fatty acids (SCFA). Commonly, the modern Western diet consists of food that is processed, stored, transported over long distances, and low in vegetables and fiber — which means your body makes fewer SCFAs, which in turn harms the way your immune system is regulated.

The hallmark of all autoimmune diseases is inflammation, or swelling. It doesn't matter which organ is affected; inflammation occurs. Autoimmune diseases can occur in any organ or tissue in your body. Examples include Type 1 diabetes, rheumatoid arthritis, psoriasis, multiple sclerosis, and lupus, among many others. If you have one autoimmune disease, your chances of developing a second one are higher.

A recent study showed that different strains of probiotics have greatly differing influences on your immune system. This important finding will help the medical community narrow research to specific bacteria that may be helpful for specific medical illnesses.

In this section, we look at how probiotics may affect diabetes and rheumatoid arthritis, as well as other autoimmune diseases.

Diabetes

Diabetes affects 220 million people globally and is responsible for 3.4 million deaths every year. There are several types of diabetes, including Type 1, which is an autoimmune condition; Type 2 diabetes, which occurs in adults and is often caused by lifestyle choices; and *gestational* diabetes, which occurs during pregnancy.

Preliminary data from Denmark suggests that the bacterial population in diabetics is different than that of people without the disease. This research opens up a potential role for modifying gut microflora with probiotics and prebiotics to improve health. Increasing numbers of diabetics in developed countries suggests that environmental factors contribute as well.

Several mice experiments using *Lactobacillus casei* showed that mice given probiotics had a smaller chance of developing diabetes. And a Finnish study on gestational diabetes found that combining probiotics with dietary counseling during and immediately after pregnancy reduced the risk of diabetes in mothers and provided a "safe and effective" tool for addressing childhood obesity (see Chapter 8).

Rheumatoid arthritis

In *rheumatoid arthritis* (often called RA), your immune system attacks normal, necessary proteins for your joints. RA patients often suffer debilitating pain and deformation of joints, especially in the hands and feet.

Researchers have found that most RA patients have abnormal gut flora. In experiments with mice, probiotics with *Lactobacillus casei* slowed the progression of RA.

Research with human RA patients is still in the very early stages, but results so far appear promising. In one study, for example, 43 RA patients were divided into two groups; one ate food rich in *Lactobacilli*, and a control group ate a regular diet. After one month, stool tests showed significant diet-induced changes in fecal flora in the probiotics group, compared to the control group. The probiotics patients also reported improvement in their RA.

Another study involved giving probiotics with *Lactobacillus rhamnosus GG* to 21 RA patients over 12 months. Although there was no statistical improvement in patients' activity, they reported an improved sense of well-being.

Although research on probiotics and autoimmune diseases is still in its infancy, early results indicate that intestinal functions are often disrupted with autoimmune conditions, which changes the composition of gut flora. These changes may result in absorption of substances into the bloodstream, which may cause flare-ups of an autoimmune disease.

Probiotics seem to modify the immune system, making people less likely to develop autoimmune problems. Concrete research into many of these autoimmune diseases doesn't exist yet, but the theory that probiotics will have a positive impact is very likely valid. Stay tuned as researchers delve deeper.

Managing Weight

The obesity epidemic has millions of people looking for ways to lose weight, and some initial studies indicate taking probiotics might help support a weight-loss plan.

Studies done in mice and human beings are showing evidence that sometime in the near future, we will be using probiotics for weight management.

Researchers from the University of Tennessee showed that consuming three to four servings of dairy products a day can help you shed more pounds than cutting out dairy (a common but erroneous weight-loss tactic).

It's possible the next "big thing" in weight management may be balancing the good bacteria in the digestive system. A Stanford University study in 2008 found that probiotics helped adult gastric bypass patients lose even more weight. Probiotics were given to these patients to improve GI functioning and quality of life. But those patients lost more weight than expected.

A breakthrough article published in *Nature* magazine in 2006 reported that microbial populations in the gut are different in obese and lean people. When obese people lose weight, their gut flora changes to become like that of lean people, suggesting that obesity may have a microbial component.

Given the accumulating evidence that gut flora impacts weight, there may well be a new obesity treatment using probiotics and prebiotics on the horizon. In the meantime, many foods shown to protect against obesity (whole plant foods, fiber, prebiotics, probiotics) appear to mediate weight gain through the gut flora; see Chapter 11 for more on probiotic- and prebiotic-rich foods.

Chapter 10

Exploring the Promise of Probiotics

. . . .

In This Chapter

▶ Checking out more about probiotics and gastrointestinal health

▶ Thinking about probiotics and oral health, skin care, weight management, and more

. . . .

*T*he promise of probiotics — using good bacteria to prevent and fight disease — is beginning to overcome the mindset that all bacteria are bad. That mindset is, unfortunately, reinforced by a germophobic culture that stuffs its store shelves with anti-bacterial cleansers.

The use of probiotics and prebiotics in the medical field is growing as more evidence accumulates supporting their benefits. First accepted by the gastroenterology community, their use is spreading to pediatrics, gynecology, and other specialties.

The United States lags behind much of the rest of the world in promoting probiotics, but that's expected to change. In fact, the global probiotics market is expected to be worth $32.6 billion by 2014. Experts predict that in the next 20 years, the proportion of probiotic products and so-called *functional foods* (processed foods that combine nutrition with additional health-improving ingredients, such as live microorganisms) will reach 30 percent of the total grocery market, up from just 3 percent today. Probiotic and prebiotic products are added to store shelves daily, and that market is expected to grow at an annual rate of 20 percent for years to come. Eventually, probiotics and prebiotics will become part of a daily regimen, taken along with vitamins.

Knowing that probiotic strains work in varied ways, customized probiotics will probably hit the shelves in the next
decade. These combinations of several strains in one pill will
focus on your medical concerns, addressing, for example,
high cholesterol, anxiety issues, appetite suppression, or
colon cancer risk. Stanford University's Dr. Justin Sonnenberg
says it's theoretically possible that warding off infection,
cancer, or autoimmune diseases may someday be a simple
matter of mixing up different microbes.

Although the current focus is on gastrointestinal health, other
less-obvious probiotic products — such as probiotic chewing
gum and drinking straws and bottle caps laced with
probiotics — are either already on the market or looming on
the horizon. In this chapter, you read about these and other
exciting possibilities the future holds for probiotics products
(and therefore for your overall health).

Exploring More Gastrointestinal Uses for Probiotics

The growing use of probiotics to treat gastrointestinal problems is expected to include using supplements for prevention.
Continued increases in the incidence of antibiotic-associated
diarrhea and *C. diff* colitis (see Chapter 4) will probably lead
to a surge in probiotic rectal suppositories and enemas.

Someday you may even be able to test your own stool for bacterial composition, which could allow you to treat your body
with customized probiotics. This kind of home test will also
make it easier for consumers to see whether the probiotic
is working. Repeated stool testing will show clearly if what
you're taking is changing your gut flora and effectively treating whatever symptom or illness you're trying to treat.

Routine use with antibiotics

Scientific research strongly supports the benefits of taking
a probiotic every time you take an antibiotic. Already, many
doctors prescribe the two together, and this trend will probably continue. In fact, it will be surprising if you don't soon
find one pill that contains both an antibiotic and a probiotic.

Additional research indicates that the prebiotic oligofructose is useful in preventing recurrence of *C. diff* diarrhea, so a prebiotic may be included in the pill, especially if the patient has a history of *C. diff* in the past. (Turn to Chapter 4 for more on *C. diff* and other types of diarrhea.)

One thing the research hasn't addressed is how long you should continue taking a probiotic when you take antibiotics. Most doctors prescribe it while you're taking the antibiotic and for a few weeks afterward.

Probiotics, prebiotics, and vitamins

Creating one pill with probiotics and prebiotics — called a synbiotic — is already a growing industry. The term *synbiotics* comes from the *synergy* (an interaction that produces a result greater than the sum of its parts) between probiotics and prebiotics.

Some companies, such as New Chapter (www.newchapter. com) are beginning to add vitamins to the combination. This trend will continue, making it easy for you to add probiotics and prebiotics to your daily supplement regimen.

Some beneficial bacteria produce vitamins themselves (see Chapter 3), which adds to gut health. Adding synbiotics to their vitamin products also lets companies legitimately claim that their pills help with immunity, keeping them out of trouble with the Food and Drug Administration.

Foreign travel

International travel is common, both for work and pleasure, and so is packing a bottle of Pepto-Bismol and a prescription antibiotic. Twenty percent of people traveling to developing countries get traveler's diarrhea (see Chapter 4). Although over-the-counter medicines may reduce the likelihood of traveler's diarrhea, it can be challenging to take them four times daily (as directed) during a busy trip.

Probiotics may soon be part of every traveler's preparations, just as getting vaccinations is essential before traveling internationally. Research has shown that several probiotics (*Saccharomyces boulardii* and a mixture of *L. acidophilus* and *Bifidobacteria*) have a significant impact in preventing traveler's diarrhea.

Suppositories

Rectal suppositories and enemas containing probiotics aren't available commercially at time of this writing. Although the theory of using such a delivery method for probiotics makes sense and is similar to fecal transplantation (Chapter 4), the medical world has been slow to consider these products. There is anecdotal research that they work in patients with antibiotic-associated diarrhea, *C. diff* colitis, and ulcerative colitis.

Probiotic suppositories containing *Lactobacilli* strains to prevent and treat bacterial vaginosis and yeast infections are available now in the United States. Although their use hasn't become commonplace yet, several studies found probiotics to be effective for treating these illnesses (see Chapter 6).

Infant formulas

Probiotics and prebiotics are now being incorporated into some infant formulas. Breast feeding is still considered the gold standard of nutrition for infants, in part because it promotes intestinal microflora that is rich in *Lactobacilli* and *Bifidobacteria*.

A couple brands of infant formulas now have probiotics added to them (Enfamil PREMIUM and Nestle Goodstart Probiotic Infant Formula, for example), but probiotic and prebiotic formulas likely will be the norm in the future.

Checking out Other Uses for Probiotics

For the last two decades, probiotics have been used primarily for digestive health. But as more studies show their usefulness in prevention and treatment of a variety of diseases, the number of probiotic products for areas other than the GI system is increasing.

This section explores some of these non-GI products and looks at how they can help improve your health.

Tampons and douches

A Swedish biotech company, Ellen AB, began selling probiotic tampons in 2003 with natural fibers treated with lactic acid bacteria. They have been shown to decrease yeast and urinary tract infections in women (replacing an old household remedy of dipping a tampon in yogurt).

Probiotic douches also are making an appearance on store shelves. They are considered a safe alternative to vinegar and water douches. The probiotic versions provide both cleansing action and also help prevent and treat vaginal yeast infections. Yeast-Gard Cleansing Douche (www.yeastgard.com) is one example.

Oral health: Lozenges, mints, gum, and toothpaste

Several companies have launched products based on research that finds probiotic to be good for oral and sinus health. There are probiotic gums, such as TheraBreath Aktiv-K12 (www.therabreath.com), and lozenges such as GUM Periobalance (www.periobalance.com).

Oragenics (www.oragenics.com) sells ProBiora3, a patented blend of three beneficial bacteria naturally present in healthy mouths, including *Streptococcus oralis* KJ3, *Streptococcus uberis* KJ2, and *Streptococcus rattus* JH145. Their products include mints, a chewable for kids, and even a powder for pets — all designed to promote fresher breath, whiter teeth, and healthy gums and teeth.

Probiotic lozenges may reduce levels of three different pathogens if you have *chronic periodontitis* (the most common type of gum disease), according to a study published in the *Journal of Oral Microbiology*. The probiotic *L. reuteri* inhibits plaque formation and decreases bleeding from gums.

Probiotic toothpastes also are hitting the U.S. market, including Design for Health's PerioBiotic Toothpaste and OMX Toothpaste. Expect to see more of these products. In addition, you can buy probiotic mouthwash, such as Compete50 Probiotic Mouthwash and KForce Balance Rinse. A Swedish study found that rinsing with a probiotic-enhanced mouthwash reduced disease-causing pathogens in the upper respiratory tract, possibly reducing respirator-related pneumonia.

Skin care

Medical literature is beginning to show that changing the gut flora can help with a variety of skin problems, such as psoriasis, eczema, dandruff, skin rashes, and rosacea. Skin care is a relatively new market for probiotic products because until recently topical probiotic applications weren't feasible. Now, though, the technology has advanced, and major players are involved.

For example, the SK1N Probiotics Online Store (www. sk1Nprobiotics.com) says its advanced line of skin products provides long-term benefits for treating some of the skin issues listed earlier. Other products on the market include Epicuren Acidophilus Probiotic Facial Cream, certain Clinique makeup and cleansers, and skin brighteners from Miessence.

Straws and bottle caps

Probiotic straws are new on the market; the probiotic is suspended in an oil droplet in the straw. They're designed primarily for use with children. Biogaia's straw contains *L. Reuteri*, a natural *Lactobacillus* that helps the beneficial bacteria restore a natural balance in your gut. *L. Reuteri* has been tested in a number of clinical studies and has been shown to be safe and effective.

In 2009, Ganeden Biotic introduced a probiotic cap dispensing system, where probiotics are stored in the bottle cap. In addition to probiotics, the cap also contains antioxidants from fruit concentrates, vitamins, and prebiotic fibers. Global Harvest, a U.S. company, and Starone Group of Frankfurt both have patented bottle caps that keep the product separate from the liquid until it's dispensed into the drink when the cap is twisted.

Treating anxiety

Prescription medications for treating anxiety have proliferated over the last few decades. Homeopathic supplements also have been popular, and now it seems as if probiotics may be taking their place in the market.

A study from a Canadian probiotics group found a significant decrease in anxiety with the use of probiotics. They attributed their findings to boosting mood-elevating chemicals in your body such as tryptophan (an amino acid) and serotonin (a neurotransmitter). A Yale University study on mice also showed that when the gut flora was altered, there was a difference in brain development and anxious behaviors. Another study found that supplements of *L. casei Shiroto* may ease anxiety symptoms in people with Chronic Fatigue Syndrome.

Recent evidence suggests that probiotics can exert beneficial effects on your psychological wellbeing as well as on your physical health. Mark Lyte, professor at Texas Tech University's School of Pharmacy, has proposed that probiotics produce neurochemicals that improve psychological health. Essentially, probiotics like *Lactobacillus* and *Bifidobacteria* produce neurochemicals in the gut that circulate through the bloodstream and induce behavioral changes.

A French study of probiotics showed potential in their use to help stress-related conditions. *Lactobacillus casei* improved mood scores in normal subjects and decreased anxiety in subjects with Chronic Fatigue Syndrome.

Given such studies, you'll likely see probiotic formulas targeted at reducing anxiety in the not-too-distant future.

Weight management

The obesity epidemic encourages millions of people to look for ways to lose weight, and some initial studies indicate that taking probiotics might help support a weight-loss plan.

A breakthrough article published in *Nature* magazine in 2006 reported that microbial populations in the gut are different in obese and lean people. When obese people lose weight, their gut flora changes to become like that of lean people, suggesting that obesity may have a microbial component.

Given the accumulating evidence that gut flora impacts weight, a new obesity treatment using probiotics and prebiotics may well be on the horizon. In the meantime, many foods shown to protect against obesity (whole plant foods, fiber, pre-biotics, probiotics) appear to mediate weight gain through the gut flora; see Chapter 11 for more on probiotic- and prebiotic-rich foods.

Aging and wellbeing

In the early 20th century, Elie Metchnikov became curious about the diet of Bulgarian peasants because of their long life, eventually discovering probiotics (see Chapter 1). Clearly, probiotics have some implications for aging well.

Doctors know that the numbers of *Lactobacilli* and *Bifidobacteria* in your gut decrease with age. In addition, your immune system becomes weaker as you get older (which is why senior citizens are strongly urged to get flu shots every year). Probiotics and prebiotics may boost those decreasing bacteria in the gut and in turn boost the immune system. The stronger the immune system is, the less likely elderly people are to succumb to illnesses that often cause serious problems. The specific mechanics are still to be explored, but there's little doubt the fermented foods in their diet kept those Bulgarian peasants young!

Part III
Adding Probiotics to Your Lifestyle

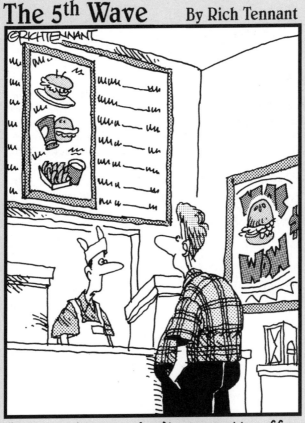

The 5th Wave   By Rich Tennant

"Sorry sir – we don't currently offer an 'Acidophilus Burger.'"

In this part . . .

With a thorough understanding of probiotics and prebiotics and how they can benefit your health, the next challenge is seeing how you can incorporate these healthful bacteria into your life. In this section, I explore ways to increase the amount of probiotics and prebiotics found in what you eat. That means some delicious recipes — appetizers, main dishes, desserts — that include fermented foods like yogurt and kefir.

Chapter 11

Filling Your Diet with Probiotics

*P*robiotic-rich foods contain live, beneficial bacteria. Incorporating these foods into your daily diet is an easy way to make sure you reap the benefits of good bacteria. There's nothing new about this: Before refrigeration, *fermentation* — adding bacteria or yeast to foods, which causes a chemical breakdown — prolonged the shelf life of foods such as cabbage (sauerkraut) and milk (yogurt).

In this chapter, you discover how to get the most out of the food on your plate by adding probiotic-rich choices to your diet. Of course, probiotics work best when they're combined with prebiotics — the stuff probiotics live on (see Chapter 2) — so I also cover prebiotic-rich foods. Finally, this chapter explores your options with probiotic supplements and offers an understanding of how to figure out the proper dose for your needs.

Identifying Probiotic-Rich Foods

The buzz phrase now in the food industry is *functional foods*, meaning that manufacturers add beneficial products to foods to encourage customers to buy them. They might add bacteria (probiotics), vitamins, or antioxidants.

Probiotic foods contain a variety of bacteria. The most common include:

- *Lactobacillus acidophilus*
- *L. bulgaricus*
- *L. casei*
- *L. johnsonii*
- *L. reuteri*
- *Bifidobacterium lactis*
- *B. breve*
- *B. infantis*
- *B. longum*
- *Streptococcus thermophilus*

See Table 11-1 for bacteria commonly found in certain foods.

Table 11-1   Bacteria Commonly Found in Foods

Food	Bacteria
Yogurt	*Lactobacillus bulgaricus*, *Streptococcus thermophilus*, *Lactobacillus acidophilus*, and various *Bifidobacteria*
Cheese	*Lactobacilli* strains
Kefir	*Lactobacilli* and *Bifidobacteria*
Pickles, sauerkraut, miso, kimchi	*Lactobacilli*

If a label reads "contains live (or active) cultures," you can look at the ingredient list to see which bacteria are in the product. Some food products contain probiotics simply because of their manufacturing process (such as sauerkraut).

In the following sections, I look at some foods that either have probiotics added by the manufacturer or contain probiotics naturally.

Going dairy: Yogurt, kefir, and other dairy products

Yogurt is the best-known food for probiotics. Thanks to excellent marketing, many yogurt companies have taken the lead in educating the public about the benefits of probiotics.

The U.S. Food and Drug Administration requires that any product called "yogurt" must contain *Lactobacillus bulgaricus* and *Streptococcus thermophilus*. But that doesn't mean those products contain the *live* cultures that are necessary to get probiotic benefits. Check the label to make sure the product contains live cultures.

Even though U.S. yogurts contain *L. bulgaricus* and *S. thermophilus*, manufacturers often add other bacteria such as *Lactobacillus acidophilus* and *Bifidobacteria*.

Unfortunately, some yogurt companies *pasteurize* (heat) the yogurt after the cultures are added, which kills the good bacteria as well as the bad. Look at the label or the company's website to see whether cultures are added before or after pasteurization. If the label specifies "live cultures," that means the cultures were added after pasteurization.

When sweeteners and flavors are added to yogurt, they may reduce the probiotic effects of live cultures. Homemade yogurt is an alternative. In India, people commonly end a meal with homemade yogurt to help with digestion. See the nearby sidebar, "How to make homemade yogurt," for an easy and probiotic-rich alternative to store-bought yogurts.

Several other dairy products contain naturally occurring probiotics or are fortified with probiotics. The following foods are some examples:

- ✔ **Buttermilk:** Buttermilk is the sour liquid left over when cream or whole milk is churned for butter. Manufacturers also make buttermilk by adding microorganisms to sweet milk. Either way, buttermilk contains probiotics.

- ✔ **Cheese:** The longer cheese is aged, the higher the probiotic content. Some manufacturers add probiotics; Kraft LiveActive cheese products, for example, contain *B. lactis* and *L. rhamnosus*.

> ✔ **Kefir:** This fermented milk drink has cultures made from various lactic acid bacteria and also the yeast *Sacchromyces*. Kefir, now available in the organic dairy section of many grocery stores, usually contains more strains of bacteria than yogurt, but has a lower total bacterial count gram-for-gram.

Finding fermentation: Sauerkraut, miso, pickles, and more

Fermentation can create probiotic-rich foods. However, sometimes modern processing can kill the probiotics, so you need to read labels carefully.

Examples of nondairy probiotic-rich foods include:

> ✔ **Sauerkraut:** Sauerkraut is fermented cabbage, created by allowing cabbage to sit, which increases the lactic acid bacteria (which are in the air) in the food. Commercial sauerkraut manufacturers sometimes kill the helpful bacteria during processing; buy only brands that specify "uncooked" on the label.

> Sauerkraut is easy to make! Turn to Chapter 12 for recipes for this food and many others that incorporate probiotics and prebiotics. *Kimchi* is a spicy Korean version of sauerkraut, also made from fermented cabbage. One study of kimchi found 31 strains of *Lactobacilli*.

> ✔ **Miso:** Miso is a fermented Japanese seasoning made from various beans and grains and used as a sauce, spread, or in soups. Add it to a hot dish only after you're done cooking it; heat kills probiotics.

> ✔ **Pickles:** Pickles, or cucumbers fermented in vinegar, contain probiotics as long as they aren't pasteurized. The pasteurization process kills probiotics.

> ✔ **Microalgae:** Microalgae supplements are made from ocean-based plants such as spirulina and blue-green algae.

> ✔ **Tempeh:** A high-protein soy product, tempeh has the chewy texture of meat. Unlike tofu, which is made from soybean milk, tempeh uses fermented whole soybeans. You can find tempeh at health food stores.

How to make homemade yogurt

Making homemade yogurt could hardly be easier. Bring some milk to a boil, just to the point where it begins to froth, on the stovetop or in the microwave. (The amount of milk you use is the amount of yogurt you'll have in the end. We typically use a half gallon of milk.)

Let cool until lukewarm and add 1 teaspoon of yogurt containing live bacteria. You can buy yogurt with live cultures at the store, use a yogurt culture starter, or borrow a yogurt starter from another family who makes yogurt.

Mix the yogurt culture into the milk, then cover and let stand somewhere warm. (My family makes yogurt every evening. We leave it sitting overnight in the microwave, which seems to retain heat.)

You'll have yogurt the next morning!

Finding Prebiotic-Rich Foods

Prebiotics are fibers that help probiotics thrive and multiply. The standard American diet — full of processed foods, sugar, and low in fiber — is lacking in prebiotics.

Prebiotic-rich foods include oats, chicory, banana, garlic, and onions, all of which contain inulin. Other foods rich in prebiotics include raw chicory root, raw Jerusalem artichoke, raw dandelion greens (each of which are 25 percent prebiotics by weight), as well as raw leeks, raw asparagus, raw wheat bran, whole wheat flour, artichokes, barley, legumes, beans, flax seed, and oats.

Look for prebiotics in the ingredient list, usually listed as *inulin* and *oligofructose*. Other prebiotics to look for include *fructooligosaccharides* (FOS), *galactooligosaccharides* (GOS), *xylooligosaccharides* (XOS), *lactulose*, and *polydextrose*.

Supplementing Your Diet

The foods you eat impact your health, and not just by controlling weight, which is the first thing most people consider.

What you choose to put in your body — from sugars to preservatives to fruits and veggies — makes a difference to your health and lifestyle on many levels.

Fortunately, many foods containing probiotics are healthy for you, making it easy to blend them into your diet.

Even though probiotic-rich foods are healthful choices, you probably need probiotic supplements to ingest *enough* bacteria to make a difference. Supplements are especially important if you're treating a specific illness, such as inflammatory bowel disease (see Chapter 2) or other health issues.

The following sections explore how probiotic supplements are made, what to look for when choosing a supplement, and how to decide on the proper dose.

Understanding how probiotics are made

The first probiotics were manufactured through fermentation, which was used to extend the shelf life of food. Kefir, for example, was fermented by adding kefir seeds to milk that was stored in a bladder and hung in the doorway. When people went through the door, they jostled the bladder, mixing the kefir and promoting the fermentation process.

Modern production isn't too dissimilar from the traditional way of making kefir. In place of bladders, companies use large fermentation vessels that maintain an optimal temperature for whatever bacteria is being grown. In place of milk, manufacturers use milk substitutes that contain many milk components like proteins, lipids (fats), and carbs.

Bacterial cultures have to be grown in the proper medium to ensure abundant quantities. No manufacturer will tell you exactly what fermentation media they use because that's the key to their business success (just as Coke or Pepsi wouldn't give away their secret formulas). The *media* is what the bacteria develop in — the "secret sauce" that grows the good bacteria. A lot of research goes into selecting growth media. When bacterial growth reaches the expected concentration levels, the product is harvested or removed from the medium. A centrifuge — a machine that spins like a big merry-go-round — separates the bacteria from the growth medium. Then the probiotics are freeze-dried before being packaged. Freeze-drying removes moisture and puts the bacteria in a state of suspended animation, which extends the bacteria's life.

Choosing a probiotic supplement

Even people in the medical profession would be at a loss in the supplements aisle of the grocery store or shopping online for probiotics. Because the research is still in its infancy, specific recommendations about how much good bacteria you should take (or, in some cases, which strain will help particular diseases or health conditions) just aren't available. However, here are some points to keep in mind:

- ✔ **What goes in your mouth doesn't necessarily reach your colon.** Good bacteria can't help you if they don't survive your stomach acid. Look for products labeled "encapsulated" or some other indication that they use technology to help the good bacteria reach your colon.

- ✔ **More strains of bacteria are better than one.** Make sure your supplement includes *Lactobacillus* and *Bifidobacteria* strains. Also check for prebiotic ingredients like *inulin*; prebiotics make the probiotic bacteria more effective. (Probulin is a good example of this kind of supplement.)

The more strains of bacteria in the supplement you take, the better. For example, Probulin has several types of bacteria. Single-strain formulations are less effective. No one's sure how many strains is the perfect number, but researchers do know that "more is better" when it comes to probiotics.

- ✔ **Always check the expiration date and storage information.** Some supplements need to be chilled; even those that don't require refrigeration should be stored away from heat.

Heat destroys probiotic bacteria, so don't drink coffee, hot tea, or other hot beverages for an hour after you take probiotics in any form — either as a supplement or in foods.

Deciding on the right dose

To promote general good health, take between 1 billion and 3 billion CFUs (colony-forming units) per day. Just as with the number of bacterial strains, more is better with CFUs too.

In recent years, several studies of probiotic products found the products didn't contain as many bacteria as the manufacturer claimed on the label. Presumably, bacteria are lost somewhere in the process during manufacturing, shipping, or storage. The bacterial concentration at the time of consumption — not at the time of manufacture — is what matters. You're dealing with live bacteria, and the longer they're alive, the better! Unfortunately, it's difficult for the consumer to be sure of the manufacturing process. Read the label carefully because many products offer assurances on their production processes.

If you're dealing with an illness, you should take at least 5 billion to 10 billion CFUs per day. Always increase your probiotics when taking antibiotics and for one to two weeks after you stop taking antibiotics to help combat the side-effects of antibiotics (see Chapter 4). Finally, if you travel abroad, up your dose of probiotics beginning two weeks before your trip and during your travels to maintain gastrointestinal health.

When you're treating a particular illness, do a little bit of research online or talk to your doctor to help you determine specific bacterial strains that may help your health problem. For instance, when it comes to allergies, studies have found *L. planatum*, *L. rhamnosus*, *L. casei*, and *L. bulgaricus* have shown positive results. (Chapters 4 through 8 all address specific health conditions.)

Looking at contraindications

Although probiotics have an excellent safety record, they should be used with caution in babies born prematurely and in people with immune deficiencies, such as transplant patients and people with HIV. If you're taking immunosuppressive drugs or chemotherapy, consult with your doctor before taking probiotics.

Some studies have found that *Lactobacillus* strains may be an issue with people who are extremely sensitive to milk or lactose. Other concerns have been raised about *S. boulardii* affecting patients with yeast allergies. Consult your physician.

Using Probiotic Snacks and Drinks

As medical science has begun to research and recognize the positive contributions probiotics make to your diet, the business community is paying attention to the trend. The United States is a little behind in the world market, but one market report suggests the global probiotics market will be worth $32.6 billion by 2014.

As companies move to grab a slice of this market, your local health food and conventional grocery stores will add a plethora of probiotics products to their shelves. Products you may encounter include:

- **Probiotic "shots":** Popular in other countries, these drinks are newly arrived in the United States. Look for DanActive (*L. casei*), Activia (*Bifidus regularis*), GoodBelly (*L. plantarum* and *B. lactis*), and Yakult (*L. casei shirota*). Other probiotic drinks include kefir beverages from Lifeway and BodyEcology; some fruit juices also now have probiotics.

- **Probiotic snacks:** ShaSha Bread Co.'s buckwheat snacks contain prebiotics and probiotics (*inulin* is the prebiotic, and *Bacillus coagulans* is the probiotic). Other probiotic snacks include Kraft LiveActive granola bars and Attune chewy chocolate and peanut butter and chocolate granola bars.

- **Probiotic chocolate:** Youngevity (`www.youngevity.com`) Triple Treat Chocolate encapsulates *L. helveticus* and *B. longum* so they aren't destroyed by the stomach acid. Ganeden Labs and Agostoni Chocolate have partnered to make several private-label chocolates with Ganeden's patented BC30 probiotic; the chocolates are available at a variety of health food and nutrition stores and may even be available at your local grocer.

- **Kombucha:** A tart and tangy beverage made from fermented tea, kombucha is a great vegan source of probiotics. BAO (`www.drinkbao.com`) makes BAO FRESH kombucha drinks, which are a slightly fizzy alternative to unhealthy sodas.

✔ **Naked Pizza:** Naked Pizza (www.nakedpizza.biz) puts probiotics, including Ganeden BC30, in its crust and other ingredients.

Looking at Other Probiotic Products

Probiotics aren't just for food. They're showing up in an ever-expanding range of products, from suppositories and enemas to facial cleansers (such as Clinique's Probiotic Cleanser) and pet products. Even sunblock lotions and drinking straws are made with probiotics these days.

In 2003, the Swedish biotech company Ellen AB began selling probiotic tampons treated with lactic acid bacteria. The tampons decrease yeast and urinary tract infections in women.

Other products with probiotics include:

✔ Gum for oral and teeth health (www.profreshmints.com)

✔ Face creams (such as Epicuren acidophilus probiotic cream)

✔ Soaps (Dr. Ohhira's Probiotic Kampuku soap)

✔ Makeup (Clinique SPF 15)

✔ Anti-aging serums (Bioelements)

✔ Skin brighteners (Miessence)

Chapter 12

Cooking Up Delicious Probiotic-Rich Meals

*T*his chapter contains some great recipes from the book *Wild Fermentation,* by Sandor Katz; delicious recipes from author Tracy Olgeaty Gensler, who wrote *Probiotic and Prebiotic Recipes for Health: 100 Recipes that Battle Colitis, Candidiasis, Food Allergies, and Other Digestive Disorders;* and also recipes from Topeka, Kansas, cook Jaya Challa. In addition, Donna Gates, creator of the first probiotics diet, generously shared many of her recipe ideas found on www. bodyecology.com. Her Body Ecology Diet re-introduces fermented, probiotic-rich foods into the modern diet.

Fermented foods have been a part of most diets for thousands of years. Today, with modern preservation methods available, many people don't have fermented foods in their diet. The process of fermenting is remarkably easy and is a great way to add probiotics to your diet.

Fermenting with Whey: Sweet Potato Fly

Prep time: *30 minutes* • **Fermentation time:** *3 days* • **Yield:** *1 gallon*

1 teaspoon/5 milliliters powdered mace

2 large sweet potatoes

2 cups/500 milliliters sugar

½ cup/125 milliliters whey

2 lemons

Cinnamon

Nutmeg

1 eggshell

1   Boil 1 cup (250 milliliters) of water with mace. Remove from heat and allow to cool.

2   Grate the sweet potatoes, and rinse well through a strainer to remove starch.

3   In a large bowl, combine the grated sweet potatoes, 1 gallon (4 liters) of water, sugar, whey, the juice and grated peel of the lemons, and a pinch each of nutmeg and cinnamon.

4   Crush the cleaned eggshell into the mixture. The recipe that inspired me called for folding in stiff beaten egg whites at this point; I don't eat raw eggs so I didn't try it, but it sounds intriguing, doesn't it?

5   Add the cooled boiled mace.

6   Stir, cover to keep flies and dust out, and leave in a warm spot to ferment for about 3 days.

7   Strain into a jug, bottles, or jars, refrigerate, and enjoy.

Source: Sandor Katz, author of Wild Fermentation.

Per serving: *Calories 122 (From Fat 1); Fat 0g; Cholesterol 0 mg; Sodium 3mg; Carbohydrate 31g (Dietary Fiber 1g); Protein 0g. per 1 cup serving.*

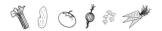

Vinagre de Piña
(Mexican Pineapple Vinegar)

Fermentation time: *3-4 weeks* • ***Yield:*** *1 quart/1 liter*

¼ cup/60 milliliters sugar

Peel of 1 pineapple (organic, because you use the skin; overripe fruits are fine)

Water

1   In a jar or bowl, dissolve the sugar in 1 quart (1 liter) of water. Coarsely chop and add the pineapple peel. Cover with cheesecloth to keep flies out, and leave to ferment at room temperature.

2   When you notice the liquid darkening, after about 1 week, strain out the pineapple peels and discard.

3   Ferment the liquid 2 to 3 weeks more, stirring or agitating periodically, and your pineapple vinegar is ready.

Courtesy of Sandor Katz, author of Wild Fermentation, *inspired by a recipe in* The Cuisines of Mexico *by Diana Kennedy*

Per serving: *Calories 6 (From Fat 0); Fat 0g; Cholesterol 0mg; Sodium 0mg; Carbohydrate 2g (Dietary Fiber 0g); Protein 0g. per 1 oz serving.*

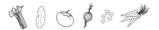

Kimchi

Fermentation time: 2 hours

2 red jalapenos (chopped)

1 green jalapeno (chopped)

4-5 garlic cloves

1 tablespoon of sugar

2 tablespoons of ginger (chopped)

1 teaspoon of red pepper flakes

2 tablespoons of fish sauce

½ head of Napa cabbage

4-6 scallions

½ cup of salt

Water

1   Cut the cabbage into 3-4 sections.

2   Fill a large container with water and dissolve the salt in it. Put the cut cabbage in the water/salt blend, making sure it's submerged. Keep at room temperature for at least 2 hours.

3   In a food processor, add chopped jalapenos (red and green), garlic cloves, sugar, chopped ginger, red pepper flakes, fish sauce, and salt to taste. Blend until it is like a paste.

4   After at least 2 hours, drain the cabbage and mix with paste. Garnish with scallions and serve cold.

Recipe courtesy of Jaya Challa

Per serving: *Calories 27 (From Fat 1); Fat 0g; Cholesterol 0mg; Sodium 1,054mg; Carbohydrate 6g (Dietary Fiber 1g); Protein 1g. per 8 oz. serving.*

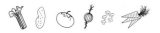

Sauerkraut

Fermentation time: 4-5 weeks

3-4 pounds of green cabbage (shredded)

3 tablespoons pickling salt

1 quart of water

1   In large mixing bowl, mix cabbage thoroughly with salt. Let stand for 20 minutes.

2   Put the cabbage mixture down into a plastic food container or even a crock pot. Pack it as tightly as possible.

3   Place a smaller lid or plate inside the container or crock pot. Weigh it down with a large glass of water.

4   Put in a dark and cool place for at least 18-24 hours. (By end of the day, the cabbage should release water and cover the cabbage.)

5   Check the container every few days for 2 weeks. You may see "scum" or mold, just wash the lid or plate that is placed on top of the sauerkraut and the glass of water and scrape away the mold you do see. (Don't worry, it is a normal occurrence.)

6   Let it stand for another 2-3 weeks.

7   Transfer to an airtight container and refrigerate.

Recipe courtesy of Jaya Challa

Per serving: *Calories 17 (From Fat 2); Fat 0g; Cholesterol 0mg; Sodium 1,340mg; Carbohydrate 4g (Dietary Fiber 2g); Protein1 g. per ½ cup serving*

Vary It! *Use red cabbage and green cabbage for pink sauerkraut. Try adding 1 tablespoon juniper berries and 2 teaspoons of caraway seeds. Add grated carrots for a coleslaw-like sauerkraut. Mix in sliced apples for a sweeter sauerkraut.*

Fermented Almond Hummus

Fermentation time: 12 hours

1 cup soaked organic almonds

1 clove garlic

Juice of ½ lemon

2 tablespoons coconut kefir or fermented vegetable juice to use as starter

Organic olive oil

Celtic sea salt to taste

1   Soak your organic almonds in a covered glass jar or bowl overnight, then rinse and blend together with lemon juice and garlic. You may want to add a small amount of water to get a creamy consistency.

2   Once blended, transfer to a sterile glass jar, add starter (either coconut kefir or fermented vegetable juice), seal tightly and let ferment at room temperature for about 12 hours.

3   Add sea salt, olive oil, and stir and then set in the fridge to chill before serving.

4   Serve with cut vegetables, lettuce wraps, or raw or baked nut, seed, or veggie crackers.

Recipe courtesy of www.bodyecology.com

Per serving: *Calories 137 (From Fat 113); Fat 13g; Cholesterol 0mg; Sodium 131mg; Carbohydrate 4g (Dietary Fiber 2g); Protein 4g. per 8 servings.*

Butternut Squash and Potato Mash Recipe

Yield: *6-8 servings*

1 large butternut squash (approximately 2 pounds), halved length-wise and seeded

1 pound potatoes, any kind, peeled or unpeeled

1 tablespoon sea salt

4 tablespoons unsalted raw butter (raw, when possible)

1 tablespoon chopped fresh rosemary

1 teaspoon chopped fresh thyme

1   Preheat oven to 400 F.

2   Place squash cut side down on baking sheet.

3   Pour 1 cup water in bottom of pan, and place in oven to roast 40-45 minutes until flesh of squash is tender when pierced with a fork. Remove from oven, and set aside.

4   Steam or boil potatoes, and add 1 teaspoon salt. When tender, remove from heat and drain.

5   When squash is just cool enough to touch, scoop flesh from skin, and combine with potatoes.

6   Melt butter in small sauté pan, and add rosemary and thyme. Simmer approximately 1 minute until herbs release aroma.

7   Add butter, herbs, and remaining salt to squash and potatoes.

8   Use either electric beater or potato masher, and mash all ingredients together until they are smooth and well combined. You may choose to leave it chunky if you are leaving skins on the potatoes. Serve warm.

Recipe courtesy of www.bodyecology.com

Per serving: *Calories 172 (From Fat 70); Fat 8g; Cholesterol 20mg; Sodium 394mg; Carbohydrate 26g (Dietary Fiber 6g); Protein 2g.*

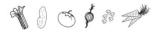

Claire's Classy Carrots Recipe

About 8 medium organic carrots

2 tablespoons ghee (clarified butter) or organic butter

Approximately ¼ cup fresh, finely chopped parsley

¼ to ½ teaspoon orange flavoring (Frontier is a good brand). If you happen to have an orange, a pinch or two of grated orange peel is a nice touch

1 drop (or to taste) stevia liquid concentrate

teaspoon (or to taste) fresh-squeezed lemon juice

1   Wash carrots and trim the ends. Cut each carrot lengthwise and then cut diagonally at about ½ inch intervals.

2   Place carrots in pan and cover with filtered water. Cover pan and cook to desired tenderness.

3   Drain carrots and set aside.

4   Place ghee or organic butter in empty carrot pan and melt on low heat. Add the orange flavoring, grated orange peel and stevia to taste.

5   Place the carrots back in the pan and toss in the orange butter. Turn off the heat, add the parsley and lemon juice, toss again and serve immediately.

Recipe courtesy of www.bodyecology.com

Per serving: *Calories 122 (From Fat 51); Fat 6g; Cholesterol 15mg; Sodium 83mg; Carbohydrate 16g (Dietary Fiber 4g); Protein 2g. per 4 servings.*

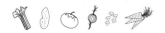

Raita

1 ½ cup plain yogurt

1 teaspoon sour cream

1 cucumber (skinless, seedless, and diced)

1 tomato (diced)

1 tablespoon cilantro

½ red onion (diced finely)

1 teaspoon of pomegranate (optional)

Pinch of ground black pepper and cumin powder

Salt to taste

1   Whisk yogurt and spoonful of sour cream until creamy. If it remains thick and stiff, thin it with a teaspoon or more of water or milk and continue whisking.

2   Stir in ALL diced vegetables and salt and pepper to taste.

3   To garnish top with finely chopped cilantro and pomegranate.

Recipe courtesy of Jaya Challa

Per serving: *Calories 51 (From Fat 22); Fat 2g; Cholesterol 9mg; Sodium 126mg; Carbohydrate 5g (Dietary Fiber 1g); Protein 3g. per 6 servings.*

Vary It! *Homemade yogurt tends to be sour; if it is, add a little bit of milk. You can use only cucumbers, or even just onions and tomatoes. Try this recipe with finely chopped mint or pineapple. To add extra seasoning to the yogurt, heat up tea oil and cumin seeds and 1/2 of a grated garlic (good antioxidant) and 1 teaspoon of cilantro. Mix with Raita.*

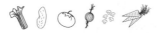

Another Delicious Cultured Veggie Recipe

1 head green cabbage, shredded in a food processor

1 bunch kale, chopped very finely by hand

5 or 6 collard leaves chopped very finely by hand

½ head cauliflower, broken in tiny florets, or chopped very, very small

2 to 3 carrots, shredded in a food processor

2 to 3 cloves garlic, peeled and minced

1 tablespoon celery seeds

1 tablespoon dried oregano

½ tablespoon dried basil

1 Using a starter culture to ensure a perfect and potent product, dissolve a package of Body Ecology Veggie Starter Culture in ¼ cup warm (90 degrees F) filtered water.

2 Add Body Ecology's EcoBloom to feed the starter if desired. You might also use a ½ tsp of Rapadura sugar or a bit of honey.

3 Let this starter mixture sit for approx. 20 minutes or longer while the L. Plantarum and other bacteria wake up and begin enjoying the sugar.

4 Add this starter culture to the brine in step 9 below.

5 Begin preparing vegetable mixture.

6 Combine all veggies, seeds, and herbs in a very large bowl.

7 Remove approx ½ of the above mixture and put into a blender.

8 Add enough filtered water to blender to create a "brine" the consistency of thick juice.

9 Blend well, then add starter culture above to this brine.

10 Add brine with culture back into veggies, celery seeds, and herbs from step one.

11 Mix together well. Note: If your blender is small you may have to do two batches but you only need to add the starter culture once.

12 Pack mixture down into as many pint or quart sized glass jars as necessary to hold all the mixture. Use a potato masher or your fist to pack veggies very tightly. You want to force out most of the air.

13 Fill container almost full, but leave about 2 inches of room at the top for veggies to expand.

14 Roll up several outer cabbage leaves into a tight "log" and place them on top to fill the remaining 2-inch space. Clamp jar closed, or screw on lid very tightly.

16 Let veggies sit at approx 70 degrees F or room temperature for at least a week. Two weeks may be even better. Refrigerate to slow down fermentation.

17 Veggies will keep in the fridge for many weeks, becoming softer and more delicious as time passes!

18 Eat at least 1/2 cup of cultured veggies with every meal and . . . enjoy!

Recipe courtesy of www.bodyecology.com

Per serving: *Calories 64 (From Fat 6); Fat 1g; Cholesterol 0mg; Sodium 54mg; Carbohydrate 14g (Dietary Fiber 5g); Protein 4g. per 8 servings.*

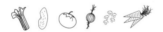

Sweet Whipped Cream Recipe

Yield: 2 cups

⅛ teaspoon white stevia powder

1 pint whipping cream

1 Place the cream in a large mixing bowl and beat with a whisk or an electric hand-held mixer until it begins to thicken.

2 Sprinkle the stevia over the cream and continue to beat until soft peaks form (do not overbeat).

3 Use immediately or place in an airtight container and refrigerate up to 4 days.

Recipe courtesy of www.bodyecology.com

Per serving: *Calories 205 (From Fat 198); Fat 22g; Cholesterol 82mg; Sodium 23mg; Carbohydrate 2g (Dietary Fiber 0g); Protein 1g. per 8 servings.*

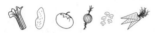

Basil Veggie Stew Recipe

1-2 tablespoons coconut oil

1 large onion, chopped

3 squirts Melissa's Basil Concentrated Extract (you can substitute 3 tablespoons dried basil, or to taste)

3 large carrots, diced into chunky pieces

3 potatoes cut about the same size as the carrots

1 cup water with sea salt

1 small head cauliflower, chopped into small florets

1 Donna loves Melissa's extracts. Not only do they add a delicious flavor, but have medicinal properties as well. In the beginning of October, they should be available at stores such as Wild Oats and even Walmart (if you can't find them in your area, call 800-588-0157). If needed, you can substitute 3 tablespoons of dried basil (or to taste).

2 In a deep skillet, sauté coconut oil, onion, and basil until it is translucent.

3 Add carrots and potatoes, continuing to saute on very low heat for 5 minutes.

4 Add 1 cup of water and sea salt. Stir well. Cover and cook on low heat for 20 minutes, until vegetables are almost tender.

5 For the last 7-10 minutes, drop in cauliflower on top of the other vegetables. Cover again. Cook until cauliflower is tender.

6 Taste and add more sea salt or Herbamare if necessary.

Recipe courtesy of www.bodyecology.com

Per serving: Calories 213 (From Fat 36); Fat 4g; Cholesterol 0mg; Sodium 342mg; Carbohydrate 42g (Dietary Fiber 8g); Protein 6g per 4 servings.

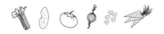

EZ Traditional Miso Soup

5-inch strip wakame (sea vegetable)

1 large onion (about 1 cup)

4 cups filtered water

2 tablespoons miso (ideally, fermented for 6 months to 2 years)

Garnish: chopped parsley, green onions, ginger, or watercress

1   Soak the wakame in water for 10 minutes and slice in into 1.5-inch pieces.

2   Thinly slice onions.

3   Put water, onions, and wakame in a saucepan and bring to a boil.

4   Reduce the heat to simmer for 10-20 minutes, until tender.

5   Remove 1.5 cups of broth from the saucepan, place in a bowl.

6   Allow water in the bowl to cool a bit and add the miso, mixing it into the water (the water should not be boiling, because it can kill the live beneficial microflora and enzymes in miso. In general, the microflora in koji, the starter used to make miso, die at 105 F).

7   Turn off heat, allow the water to cool a bit.

8   Add the miso broth to the soup in the saucepan and add chopped parsley, green onions, ginger, or watercress for garnish.

Vary It! The above recipe is a vegetarian version. You can also add bonito flakes (dried fish) — check out bonito flakes at Amazon.com or check with your local Asian market. Simmer one tablespoon of bonito flakes in the water for 10 minutes and strain. Then continue as above. When made with the dried fish as a quick stock, your miso soup will be even more strengthening.

Recipe courtesy of www.bodyecology.com

Per serving: Calories 34 (From Fat 5); Fat 1g; Cholesterol 0mg; Sodium 321mg; Carbohydrate 6g (Dietary Fiber 1g); Protein 2g per 4 servings.

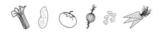

Dill-icous Cultured Beet Salad

Yield: *6-8 servings*

5 lbs red beets, shredded in food processor

3 bunches of dill

Juice of 4-5 lemons

1-2 cloves garlic

Caraway seeds to taste

About ¼ cup raw apple cider vinegar

About 12 cabbage leaves

Pure water

1 green apple

Few stalks of celery

1 Veggie culture starter from Body Ecology

Equipment: Small drinking glass, large mixing bowl, sterile mason jars

1   Empty the contents of your room temp starter culture into a 4-ounce glass of warm water and set aside.

2   Shred your beets in food processor, and then add them to mixing bowl.

3   Finely chop half of your dill and add that to mixing bowl.

4   Add caraway seeds and raw apple cider vinegar.

5   Blend 1 green apple, about 4 cups water, handful of beets, celery, garlic, lemon juice, and the remainder of dill in Vitamix or really good blender.

6   Once blended, add your water/culture starter mix to your blender and stir.

7   Pour liquid mixture over beets and mix well with large spoon.

8   Pack your sterile mason jars with these cultured vegetables, leaving about 1.5 inches at top.

9   Roll up some cabbage leaves and place atop each jar before sealing.

10 Seal each jar tightly, run under hot water, and wipe clean.

11 I always do a blessing or intention on my veggies... you can do this now if you choose.

12 Ferment for 5-10 days at room temp. The longer you ferment, the more sour they become.

By Gina LaVerde (Recipe courtesy of www.bodyecology.com)

Per serving: *Calories 146 (From Fat 6); Fat 1g; Cholesterol 0mg; Sodium 224mg; Carbohydrate 34g (Dietary Fiber 9g); Protein 5g.*

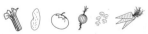

Green Bean Salad Recipe

Yield: *4 servings*

2 pounds green beans, trimmed

3 ears corn, kernels removed when raw

½ small red pepper

1 small red onion

⅓ cup chopped basil

⅛ cup extra virgin olive oil

⅛ cup grape seed oil

1 tablespoon balsamic vinegar

2 tablespoons apple cider vinegar

3 tablespoons lemon juice

1   Separately blanch corn and beans.

2   Combine in large bowl.

3   Add pepper, onions, basil, oils, vinegars, lemon juice, and garlic.

4   Season with hot sauce and sea salt and pepper.

Recipe courtesy of www.bodyecology.com

Per serving: *Calories 272 (From Fat 135); Fat 15g; Cholesterol 0mg; Sodium 19mg; Carbohydrate 35g (Dietary Fiber 10g); Protein 7g.*

Summer Spaghetti Salad

(2) 7-ounce packages Angel Hair Miracle Noodles

1 chopped red pepper

2 small chopped zucchini squash

1 small chopped yellow squash

2 handfuls chopped spinach

1 handful chopped kale leaves

1 handful chopped basil

3-4 cloves of garlic (or more, to taste)

1 tablespoon each of rosemary and thyme

Hawaiian or Celtic Sea Salt, to taste

Cracked black pepper to taste

Handful dulse flakes

Lemon juice to taste

Olive oil

Unrefined coconut oil for cooking

1   Prepare your konjaku noodles as directed on the package.

2   Rinse them lightly, place in a pasta bowl, and drizzle olive oil over them.

3   Heat your coconut oil over low heat and lightly sauté the garlic, rosemary, and thyme.

4   Gradually add in your kale until soft.

5   Turn off the heat and add in your spinach so that it wilts just a little.

6   Next, pour this mixture over the noodles and lightly mix in red peppers, zucchini, basil, dulse flakes, sea salt, and pepper.

7   Drizzle each serving with a splash of lemon juice before serving, and enjoy with your favorite probiotic beverage, or fermented, cultured vegetable blend to aid in digestion.

Recipe courtesy of www.bodyecology.com.

Per serving: *Calories 97 (From Fat 65); Fat 7g; Cholesterol 0mg; Sodium 107mg; Carbohydrate 8g (Dietary Fiber 3g); Protein 3g. based on 4 servings.*

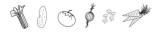

Purple & Green Cabbage Salad with Sweet & Sour Tempeh

Yield: *1 serving*

For the salad:

2 teaspoons (10 ml) sesame oil, divided

½ cup (80 g) tempeh, cubed

1 cup (155 g) pineapple chunks, fresh, or canned in juice and drained

½ cup (60 g) green pepper, thinly sliced

1 scallion, including green stem, thinly sliced

2 tablespoons (20 g) red onion, chopped

¾ cup (53 g) purple cabbage, shredded

¾ cup (53 g) green cabbage, shredded

1 cup (30 g) whole-wheat croutons

For the dressing:

2 teaspoons (10 ml) agave nectar or honey

2 tablespoons (30 ml) rice vinegar

1   To make the salad, heat 1 teaspoon (5 ml) sesame oil and the tempeh in a skillet over medium heat.

2   Sauté for 4 minutes until browned on all sides; remove from pan and drain on paper towels.

3   Add remaining 1 teaspoon (5 ml) sesame oil to the pan, then add pineapple and grill on all sides for 4 minutes. Remove from pan.

4   In a large bowl, combine peppers, scallion, onion, and cabbage. Top salad with tempeh and pineapple.

5   To make the dressing, in a small bowl, whisk together agave nectar and vinegar; pour over salad.

Recipe courtesy of Tracy Olgeaty Gensler, author of Probiotic and Prebiotic Recipes for Health: 100 Recipes that Battle Colitis, Candidiasis, Food Allergies, and Other Digestive Disorders

Per serving: *Calories 478 (From Fat 176); Fat 20g; Cholesterol 0mg; Sodium 177mg; Carbohydrate 64g (Dietary Fiber 13g); Protein 21g.*

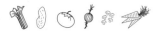

Body Ecology Turkey Loaf

Cook time: *1 hour*

1 pound ground turkey

1 egg

2 carrots, finely chopped

1 large onion, finely chopped

1 large red pepper, diced

1 ½ stalks celery, finely chopped

1 tablespoon Worcestershire sauce (we use Robbies Worcestershire made with apple cider vinegar)

1/2 teaspoon sea salt

1 tablespoon whole grain mustard

1/2 teaspoon garlic pepper powder

2 tablespoons parsley flakes

1   Combine all ingredients and mold into loaf pan.

2   Bake at 350 F for 1 hour.

Recipe courtesy of www.bodyecology.com

Per serving: *Calories 261 (From Fat 108); Fat 12g; Cholesterol 135mg; Sodium 564mg; Carbohydrate 12g (Dietary Fiber 3g); Protein 25g. per 4 servings.*

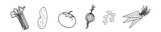

Chicken Breasts Roasted in Fresh Garden Herbs

1 cup fresh oregano leaves

1 cup green onions, coarsely chopped

4 tablespoons fresh cilantro, coarsely chopped

2 small garlic cloves

Juice of two lemons

¾ tablespoon melted coconut oil, ghee, or extra virgin olive oil

1 teaspoon fine grind celtic sea salt

½ teaspoon crushed red pepper flakes

4 free-range, organic chicken breasts

1   Combine first eight ingredients (everything but the chicken breasts) in a food processor bowl and process until minced.

2   Place chicken in a casserole dish and spread fresh herb mixture over chicken breasts.

3   Marinate chicken at least 1 hour in refrigerator then roast very slowly in a 225 F degree oven for 1 hour and 15 minutes or until the breasts are done.

Recipe courtesy of www.bodyecology.com

Per serving: Calories 237 (From Fat 69); Fat 8g; Cholesterol 73mg; Sodium 647mg; Carbohydrate 16g (Dietary Fiber 9g); Protein 29g.

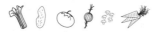

Red Bell Peppers Stuffed

Yield: *6 servings*

4 large red bell peppers, cut in half and seeded

Sea salt and pepper to taste

3 tablespoons extra virgin olive oil

1 medium yellow onion, finely chopped

2 ribs celery, finely chopped

3 cups cooked millet

¼ cup coarsely chopped fresh mint or 1 tablespoon dried

2 tablespoons finely chopped flat-leaf parsley

2 tablespoons capers, drained

3 tablespoons fresh lemon juice (about 1 lemon)

1   Sprinkle the peppers with sea salt and pepper. Preheat the oven to 400 F degrees.

2   Heat the oil in a large nonstick skillet over medium heat. Add the onion, celery, salt, and pepper. Cover and cook, stirring occasionally for about 4 minutes, or until the onion is softened.

3   Add the cooked millet, mint, parsley, capers, lemon juice, salt, and pepper. Stir to mix well. Taste for seasonings.

4   Stuff this mixture into the pepper halves. Arrange the peppers in a glass baking dish large enough to hold them in one layer. Pour 1 cup of water around, not over, the peppers.

5   Cover the pan tightly with foil.

6   Bake for about 1 hour, or until the peppers are fork-tender.

Excerpted from Invitation to Dine: Recipes from my Personal Collection, by Christiane Herzog. Recipe courtesy of www.bodyecology.com

Per serving: *Calories 206 (From Fat 71); Fat 8g; Cholesterol 0mg; Sodium 204mg; Carbohydrate 31g (Dietary Fiber 4g); Protein 5g.*

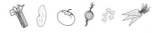

Stuffed Zucchini Boats

4-6 medium zucchini

2 cups millet, cooked

¼ cup amaranth, cooked

1 medium onion, chopped

1 medium red bell pepper, chopped

1 garlic clove, minced

¼ cup water

2-3 tablespoons coconut oil or ghee

1 teaspoon Celtic Sea Salt

1   Prepare zucchini, cut off ends, and cook whole in boiling water for approx 5-7 min.

2   Remove from water, and cut zucchini in half, lengthwise. With tip of spoon, carefully remove seeds (discard if you don't like to use the seeds), and then spoon out some of the softened zucchini. Set aside.

3   Heat oil in pan, and stir-fry onion, pepper, and garlic. When onion and pepper are half softened, add millet, amaranth, and salt to skillet with approx ¼ cup water. Add water a little bit at a time to help determine the consistency you prefer. Add softened zucchini, mix all components together, and remove from heat.

4   Spoon mixture into zucchini boats, and place in baking dish. Bake uncovered at 350 F degrees approximately 15-20 minutes or until brown on top. Enjoy this delightful seasonal favorite!

Recipe courtesy of www.bodyecology.com

Per serving: *Calories 206 (From Fat 72); Fat 8g; Cholesterol 0mg; Sodium 584mg; Carbohydrate 30g (Dietary Fiber 5g); Protein 6g.*

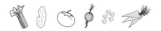

Tempeh Cubes with Ginger Vegetables

Yield: *1 serving*

1 cup (235 ml) water

½ cup (80 g) tempeh

1 tablespoon (14 g) light, trans-fat-free margarine

1 egg

½ cup (35 g) broccoli florets

2 scallions, chopped

1 teaspoon minced ginger

1 teaspoon minced garlic

1   In a small saucepan over medium-low heat, simmer the water and the tempeh for 10 minutes.

2   Remove from heat, place tempeh on several paper towels to drain; when dry, cut tempeh into cubes.

3   Melt margarine in a skillet over medium-low heat; add tempeh and sauté, stirring occasionally for 4 minutes.

4   Add egg, broccoli, scallions, garlic, and ginger and continue to sauté, stirring occasionally, for another 5 minutes.

Recipe courtesy of Tracy Olgeaty Gensler, author of Probiotic and Prebiotic Recipes for Health: 100 Recipes that Battle Colitis, Candidiasis, Food Allergies, and Other Digestive Disorders

Per serving: *Calories 353 (From Fat 224); Fat 25g; Cholesterol 212mg; Sodium 205mg; Carbohydrate 13g (Dietary Fiber 6g); Protein 23g.*

Make it a meal! *Serve over ½ cup (82 g) cooked brown rice.*

Grilled Gruyere Sandwich with Sauerkraut

Yield: *1 serving*

2 slices whole-wheat bread

1 ½ tablespoons (21 g) light, trans-fat-free margarine

1 ounce (28 g) Gruyere cheese, or fontina, sliced

⅓ cup (75 g) canned sauerkraut, drained

1   Preheat a skillet over medium heat. Spread half of the margarine on one side of one slice of bread; place bread margarine-side down in the pan.

2   Top bread with cheese and sauerkraut.

3   Spread remaining margarine on one side of the second slice of bread; place bread margarine-side up on top of sauerkraut.

4   Heat until cheese begins to melt, about 4 minutes.

5   Flip sandwich and cook the other side for 3 to 4 minutes. Slice sandwich in half to eat.

Recipe courtesy of Tracy Olgeaty Gensler, author of Probiotic and Prebiotic Recipes for Health: 100 Recipes that Battle Colitis, Candidiasis, Food Allergies, and Other Digestive Disorders

Per serving: *Calories 415 (From Fat 253); Fat 28g; Cholesterol 31mg; Sodium 881mg; Carbohydrate 28g (Dietary Fiber 5g); Protein 14g.*

Make it a meal! *Serve with 1 cup (150 g) red grapes.*

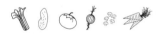

Delicious Tart Lemony Parfait with Whipped Cream

Yield: *4 servings*

6 large egg yolks, room temperature

½ cup of Lakanto that has already been finely ground in a nut grinder or VitaMix

½ cup lemon juice, freshly squeezed

1 cup water

1 heaping tablespoon agar flakes

Pinch of sea salt

6-8 drops of Body Ecology's liquid Stevia Concentrate

1 tablespoon grated lemon rind

½ cup (1 stick) unsalted butter, cut into small pieces

1   In saucepan combine eggs and Lakanto and beat together with electric beater. DO NOT HEAT YET.

2   Beat lemon juice into egg/Lakanto mixture.

3   In second saucepan bring water to a boil and add agar flakes and sea salt. Stir to dissolve and let simmer for 10 minutes. Remove from heat, but keep warm.

4   Move saucepan with egg/Lakanto/lemon juice mixture to cooktop and bring to a simmer over low heat. (Keep heat low so you do not cook the eggs.)

5   Stirring constantly, melt the butter slices into this mixture.

6   When melted, remove from heat and add lemon rind and stevia liquid concentrate.

7   Slowly pour warm agar mixture into egg/Lakanto/lemon juice/lemon rind/stevia mixing well.

8   Pour mixture into parfait glasses and let cool in refrigerator.

9   Before serving top with Lakanto or stevia-sweetened whipped cream, but only if your body is fine with dairy. Cream has casein.

Vary It! This recipe can be used as a filling to make a lemon meringue pie. For better food combining we suggest a soaked and raw nut crust for the crust and an egg white meringue.

Recipe courtesy of www.bodyecology.com

Per serving: *Calories 299 (From Fat 274); Fat 30g; Cholesterol 380mg; Sodium 49mg; Carbohydrate 4g (Dietary Fiber 0g); Protein 5g.*

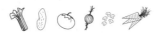

Key Lime Ice Cream

4-5 cups coconut kefir cheese

Juice of 3 limes

½ cup Lakanto

Few drops stevia (to taste)

⅛ teaspoon pure vanilla extract or vanilla bean

Pinch Celtic Sea Salt

1   In a Vitamix or food processor, combine coconut kefir cheese and lime juice, and blend for about 1 minute.

2   Add Lakanto, sea salt, and vanilla and blend for another 30 seconds.

3   Taste, and add stevia as needed.

4   Pour into freezer-safe container or ice cream maker.

5   Freeze until ready to enjoy!

Note: *If you do not have an ice cream maker, you will want to blend it once more before eating to get the creamiest consistency.*

Recipe by Gina Laverde, courtesy of www.bodyecology.com

Per serving: *Calories 90 (From Fat 42); Fat 5g; Cholesterol 0mg; Sodium 24mg; Carbohydrate 12g (Dietary Fiber 2g); Protein 1g. per 8 servings.*

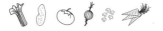

Lemon Cherry Yogurt Parfait

2 cups of young coconut kefir cheese
(coconut yogurt)

¼ cup fresh Bing cherries*

1 teaspoon agar (seaweed used like
gelatin)

3 tablespoons Lakanto

½ cup water

1 tablespoon fresh lemon juice

1 teaspoon finely grated lemon zest

Few drops of liquid stevia (to taste)

4 stemmed cherries (for topping)

4 beautiful wine glasses

1   In a food processor or high-speed blender, combine 1-cup coconut kefir cheese, Bing cherries, and a few drops of liquid stevia to taste. Blend until creamy. Move to a mixing bowl.

2   Add the remaining kefir cheese, Lakanto, lemon juice, and lemon zest to your blender and blend until creamy. Move to a separate mixing bowl.

3   Boil ½ cup of water on stovetop, turn off heat, add agar flakes, and stir until dissolved.

4   Quickly add half of the agar agar gelatin to each bowl, and stir.

5   You can re-blend each fruit/cream if you like.

6   Spoon half of the lemon cream into 4 wineglasses and top with half of the cherry cream. Top with the remaining lemon and cherry creams and refrigerate for 20 minutes before serving.

*Cherries are not included in stage one, the healing stage of Body Ecology. Sometimes even sour fruits can cause candida to act up. Ideally, fruits should be eaten alone, on an empty stomach, and combined with a good fermented food, so that the microflora can help the sugar and you can enjoy the delicious flavor.

Submitted by Travis Grant (Recipe courtesy of www.bodyecology.com)

Per serving: Calories 94 (From Fat 43); Fat 5g; Cholesterol 0mg; Sodium 7mg; Carbohydrate 13g (Dietary Fiber 2g); Protein 1g.

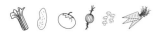

Triple Berry Sorbet

Yield: *6-8 servings*

1 pint each of strawberries, raspberries, and blueberries

Juice of 1 lemon

Liquid stevia and/or Lakanto (to taste)

2 cups coconut kefir cheese

Dash Hawaiian or Celtic Sea Salt

Splash vanilla

1   Prepare Coconut Kefir Cheese and refrigerate after it's fermented.

2   Blend berries, stevia, (or Lakanto) lemon juice, and vanilla in your Vita-Mix, and freeze in an ice cream maker or freezer safe container.

3   When ready to eat, thaw berries for a few minutes, then blend them with your kefir cheese and serve!

Recipe courtesy of www.bodyecology.com

Per serving: *Calories 122 (From Fat 33); Fat 4g; Cholesterol 0mg; Sodium 31mg; Carbohydrate 22g (Dietary Fiber 7g); Protein 1g.*

Part IV

The Part of Tens

The 5th Wave   By Rich Tennant

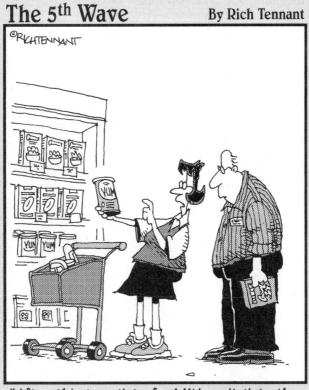

"After this long list of additives it lists the expiration date. Does that pertain to the product or the person who eats it?"

In this part . . .

In this part, I explore probiotics and prebiotics in an easy-to-understand format. I've selected the most-asked-about information and outlined it in sections that highlight ten (or so) bits of information that you need to know. Explore the impact probiotics have on allergies and asthma or scan the top ten most common questions about probiotics. It's information at your fingertips as you include probiotics in your quest to live a healthy life.

Chapter 13

Ten (Or So) Ways Probiotics Promote Good Health

*M*any benefits of probiotics are being discovered as the medical world focuses more attention on the roles of good bacteria. One thing is clear about what researchers are learning: Probiotics aren't just for digestive health. They help you with a multitude of medical conditions and with your general health, ranging from allergies to improving longevity. In fact, research is probing how probiotics may help protect against serious conditions like cancer and cardiovascular disease.

Today, people live longer than they did just a few decades ago. Probiotics are versatile in how they help you maintain your health, and they're even more crucial to your wellbeing as you age. Bacterial diversity in your gut decreases with advanced age, making you more prone to illness and disease. Probiotics can combat many of the challenges you face as you age.

Here, I summarize ten ways probiotics promote good health, whether you're using them to treat a specific condition or to just maintain your overall health.

Replenishing Good Bacteria in the Gut

More than 1,000 different strains of bacteria live in your gut, helping you digest food, synthesize vitamins, and absorb nutrients. (See Chapter 2 for more on what good bacteria do in your digestive system.)

Scientists have found that an improper balance of good and bad bacteria in your gut negatively impacts your health. In healthy individuals, the ratio of good to bad bacteria is about 10 to 1. Several factors, including environmental stress and antibiotics, are known to affect this balance, allowing bad bacteria to proliferate. Maintaining the proper ratio of good and bad bacteria is crucial for good health. Taking probiotics helps you to replenish the good bacteria and keep that critical balance.

Crowding Out Bad Bacteria

The good bacteria in probiotics push their way into your body, competing for space with the bad bacteria that can make you sick. The walls of your intestine have lots of little places, called *adherence sites,* where bacteria can "grab on." When the good bacteria latch on to those adherence sites, there is nowhere for the bad bacteria to adhere.

This isn't true only in the gut. One study found that taking *Lactobacillus acidophilus* reduced the adherence of oral *Streptococci* (the bacteria that cause strep infections, among other illnesses), reducing the risk of tooth decay.

Enhancing Your Immune System

Eighty percent of your immune system is located in your digestive system. That means your gut bacteria heavily impact the complex system in your body that protects against disease. Your body is a terrific communicator, and your gut is constantly sending messages through chemical secretions and in other ways to respond to imminent threats from bacteria, viruses, and so on.

Probiotics keep the gut bacteria in balance, which is one of the key segments of the immune system's communication. (See Chapter 3 for detailed information on how probiotics stimulate your immune system.) Research is finding that probiotics also may be useful in treating autoimmune conditions like rheumatoid arthritis and diabetes (see Chapter 9).

Much research still needs to be done on the exact mechanics of bacteria's function in immunity, but there is little doubt that good bacteria are crucial to protecting your health.

Preventing Allergies

The composition of gut flora differs in people who have allergies and those who don't. Although research is in its infancy, studies are finding a definite connection between taking probiotics and reducing allergies.

One Finnish study found that babies had 30 percent fewer incidences of eczema (which is often an early sign of allergies) when mothers were given probiotics while pregnant and babies were given probiotics for six months after birth.

Eliminating Yeast Infections

About 75 percent of women will have a yeast infection at least once in their lives. The normally acidic vaginal environment usually limits problems, but many situations can cause that environment to change — including taking antibiotics, stress, and various methods of birth control. Many studies have demonstrated that taking probiotics can reduce or eliminate yeast infections. Some U.S. doctors are beginning to prescribe probiotics along with their antibiotic prescriptions to preempt the drugs' tendency to promote yeast infections — a practice many European doctors have used for years.

L. acidophilis, *L. rhamnosus,* and *L. fermentum* have been successful in treating and preventing yeast infections.

Producing Essential Vitamins

The good bacteria in probiotics produce vitamin K2 and B vitamins, including folic acid, B12, pantothenic acid, thiamine, pyridoxine, biotin.

Vitamin K2 is important in blood clotting, and B vitamins promote energy and metabolism.

Strengthening Natural Defenses

Intestinal bacteria play an important role in providing natural defense mechanisms against invading pathogens and toxins. But the gut barrier can break down, developing "leaky gut" or increased intestinal *permeability* (the ease in which things pass through a barrier).

Probiotics cause anti-inflammatory responses in the epithelial cells, which strengthens the gut barrier and prevents bad bacteria from entering the bloodstream. These cells also contain several "signaling pathways" (see Chapter 3). Probiotics manipulate these pathways and strengthen the gut defense barrier.

In addition to being a physical barrier, probiotics can stimulate synthesis and secretion of *Immunoglobulin A,* an antibody that coats and protects mucosal surfaces from harmful bacterial invasion.

Probiotics also help your natural defense barrier by breaking down dietary sugars into short chain fatty acids, which provide a major source of energy to the epithelial cells to regenerate themselves — which keeps the barrier strong at all times.

Preventing Antibiotic-Related Diarrhea

One of the unpopular — and sometimes serious — side effects of antibiotics is diarrhea. Though it's usually just considered an inconvenience, diarrhea can cause dehydration with possible fairly dire consequences.

Antibiotics tend to kill or reduce good bacteria, thus giving bad bacteria an opportunity to grow. One of these kinds of bad bacteria is *Clostridium difficile,* commonly called *C. diff. Lactobacillus rhamnosus GG* and *Lactobacillus acidophilus* have been shown to prevent or reduce recurrences of *C. diff.* diarrhea. Many doctors now prescribe probiotics whenever they give antibiotics to prevent associated diarrhea.

Reducing Constipation, Bloating, and Diarrhea

The balance of bacteria in your gut is crucial to maintaining your digestive health. When bad bacteria multiply, the imbalance can lead to digestive upsets like constipation, bloating, and diarrhea. (See Chapter 4 for more about digestive problems.) These problems also can be caused by food, viruses, or other illnesses.

Taking probiotics helps with the symptoms of constipation, bloating, and diarrhea from a variety of causes — for example, those associated with irritable bowel syndrome and lactose intolerance. Lactose-intolerant patients who eat foods containing lactose can develop bloating and diarrhea, but many probiotics, especially the *Lactobacillus* family, contain the enzyme *lactase*, which actually digests the lactose in food, easing the symptoms of lactose intolerance.

The live cultures in fermented milk products such as yogurt contain the enzyme lactase, so even if you're intolerant to lactose, you can eat yogurt without suffering the symptoms of lactose intolerance.

Probiotics have been shown to help balance the bacteria in your digestive tract, thus helping to alleviate these common problems.

Chapter 14

Ten Misconceptions about Probiotics

*A*lthough probiotics have been around for thousands of years — and, indeed, have been used to help improve and protect health in many cultures for countless generations — their appearance on the American medical and natural health scene is relatively recent. And as with any "new big thing," some people have misconceptions about exactly what probiotics are and what they do.

In this chapter, I present ten common myths and misconceptions about probiotics, along with what scientists and health care providers know about probiotics' functions and uses in maintaining good health and preventing or treating disease.

All Bacteria Are Bad for You

The word *bacteria* elicits a basic "ick" response and an urge to wash your hands with anti-bacterial soap. But bacteria are essential to good health, and one key to understanding probiotics is dumping the idea that all bacteria are bad. Oftentimes, if it weren't for good bacteria in your digestive tract, bad bacteria would take over and make you sick.

Probiotics are good bacteria that help you by maintaining digestive health, boosting immunity, preventing urogenital infections, and controlling allergies, among other things. Initial studies even show probiotics have an impact on preventing cancer.

A Yogurt a Day Keeps the Doctor Away

You'll get no arguments from doctors that fermented dairy products like yogurt are good for you, and they're a good source of probiotics. The challenge is looking at a packed-full yogurt case at the grocery store and figuring out which product will put probiotics in your system. You need a yogurt with live cultures that were added *after* pasteurization, because the pasteurization process kills off a lot of good bacteria. (See Chapter 12 for a recipe to make your own probiotic-rich yogurt.)

However, even if you find a terrific yogurt product, you can't rely exclusively on yogurt and other foods to meet your body's probiotic needs. Even Dannon Activia yogurt, one of the national brands that adds probiotics to its products, now states in its commercials that you have to eat three servings a day to get the digestive benefits the label promises.

The foods you eat typically don't have enough probiotics to significantly impact your health. If you really want to gain the benefits of probiotics, you likely will have to take probiotic supplements. Turn to Chapter 11 for information on choosing a good probiotic supplement.

The United States Leads the World in Probiotic Use and Education

Unfortunately, although the United States leads in many medical areas, it lags far behind Europe and Asia in public education about probiotics. European doctors, for instance, regularly prescribe probiotics when they prescribe antibiotics, which helps to prevent antibiotic-related diarrhea (see Chapter 4). U.S doctors, unfortunately, don't yet routinely prescribe probiotics.

The good news is that yogurt commercials and recent advertising for probiotic products are putting probiotics in the public eye. Although many people remain unaware of the roles probiotics play in maintaining good health and recovering from or preventing illness, public awareness — and, just as important, awareness among physicians and other health care providers — is growing.

The Number of Strains in Probiotic Supplements Doesn't Matter

Medical research typically focuses on particular strains of probiotics for specific problems. The best probiotics contain multiple strains. Look for one that has several strains of *Lactobacilli* species, as well as *Bifidobacterium* species.

Your digestive system alone has more than 1,000 species of bacteria. Thus, your probiotic supplement should have multiple species and strains to really help maintain digestive health.

All Probiotic Supplements Are the Same

Unfortunately, all probiotic supplements are not created equal. When you buy a probiotic supplement, look for one with the following qualities:

- ✔ Multiple strains of probiotics
- ✔ Acid protection technology (to protect the bacteria as it travels through the acidic stomach environment)
- ✔ A high CFU count (see Chapter 11)
- ✔ Clear information on shelf life and storage instructions

What you put in your mouth doesn't necessarily reach the colon. A new generation of probiotics, such as Probulin, has specialized coatings that prevent acid destruction of the probiotics in the stomach.

Prebiotics Are an Inessential Extra

The idea that prebiotics are just window dressing for probiotics is far from the truth. As more research is done, scientists and health care providers are discovering much more about how prebiotics and probiotics work together for maximum health benefits.

Prebiotics like inulin are fuel for probiotics, helping them work better. Many companies now add prebiotics to their probiotic products precisely because of this benefit. See Chapter 3 for more about prebiotics.

You Can't Take Probiotics with Antibiotics

Antibiotics are great at killing bad bacteria that cause certain illnesses, but they can't distinguish between good and bad bacteria. As a result, many people experience bouts of diarrhea when they take antibiotics.

To help prevent antibiotic-related diarrhea, you *should* take probiotics when you take antibiotics. Doctors, particularly pediatricians, are beginning to recognize the benefits of adding probiotics to an antibiotic regimen. If your doctor doesn't mention probiotics when she prescribes antibiotics for you or a loved one, be sure to ask her whether probiotics are appropriate.

Traveler's Diarrhea Is an Unavoidable Part of Overseas Travel

For Americans, traveler's diarrhea (TD) is defined as three or more stools in a 24-hour period when you travel outside of the United States. (People who travel from other countries *to* the United States rarely get TD.) TD's symptoms usually include abdominal cramping, bloating, and occasionally nausea. The source of infection is usually ingestion of fecally contaminated food or water.

Traveler's diarrhea doesn't have to be a necessary or unavoidable part of your international travels. Studies have shown that taking probiotics before and during overseas travel can prevent TD — which will make your trip that much more enjoyable.

Probiotics May Not Be Safe for Some People

Probiotics are rated by the Food and Drug Administration as GRAS, or Generally Recognized As Safe. The GRAS designation means that probiotics generally pose no danger for most people.

However, although probiotics have an excellent safety record, they should be used with caution in babies born prematurely and in people with immune deficiencies, such as those found in HIV or with transplant patients. If you're taking immunosuppressive drugs or chemotherapy, consult with your doctor before taking probiotics.

Probiotics Don't Help the Immune System

The gastrointestinal tract is arguably the largest immune organ in the body (your skin is your largest organ and also functions as part of your immune system by protecting your body from certain contaminants). Probiotics have been shown to help strengthen your immune system by crowding out bad bacteria. Probiotics also improve the integrity of the gut lining, stopping bad bacteria from passing into your bloodstream.

Probiotics also increase the secretion of IgA antibodies, which make your immune system more powerful and effective (see Chapter 3 for more on IgA antibodies and your immune system). Although medical research about immunity and probiotics is in its infancy, initial studies indicate that probiotics help regulate and stimulate immune responses.

Chapter 15

Ten (Or So) Famous Bacteria

*E*ver since Louis Pasteur came up with germ theory in the 1860s (see Chapter 1), conventional wisdom has held that bacteria — or germs — are bad, bad, bad. Just look in the cleaning products aisle at your local grocer's and marvel at the wide range of anti-bacterial hand soaps, dish detergents, wipes, and bathroom and kitchen cleansers.

Certainly, some bacteria deserve their less-than-wholesome reputation. But many are harmless to humans, and some are beneficial. In this chapter, I take a closer look at ten well-known bacteria and discover what makes them good, bad, or downright ugly.

Bifidobacteria (Good)

The food industry and probiotics supplement manufacturers commonly use various strains of *Bifidobacteria* to enhance their products. Depending on the strain, *Bifidobacteria* support the immune system, prevent harmful bacteria from colonizing the digestive tract, and help produce vitamins and other dietary compounds your body needs.

Breast milk is high in the milk sugar *lactose*. The lactic acid bacteria in an infant's digestive tract, including *Bifidobacteria*, not only break down lactose into nutrients the baby's body can use, but also create an acidic environment that helps prevent bad bacteria from growing and causing harm.

Specific strains of *Bifidobacteria* seem to have properties that make them particularly useful or helpful. In the following sections, you discover how these common good bacteria help keep you healthy.

B. animalis

Yogurt maker Dannon uses *B. animalis* in its Activia brand of yogurt, and company-conducted studies have shown that this good bacteria survives the journey through the digestive tract (see Chapter 2) and helps regulate bowel movements.

Other studies, both related and independent, have turned up additional evidence of *B. animalis's* beneficial effects. For example, Italian researchers found that *B. animalis* helps alleviate both the symptoms and the intestinal damage associated with zinc deficiency in rats. Zinc deficiency causes ulcerations, inflammation, and other damage, but the intestinal linings in rats that received *B. animalis* were close to normal.

In humans, *B. animalis* has been shown to reduce both harmful bacteria and inflammation in the intestines.

B. breve

Bifidobacterium breve seems to fight off bad bacteria like *E. coli*. This good bacteria lives in the digestive tract and the vagina, where it helps keep bad yeast like *Candida albicans*, the primary cause of yeast infections (see Chapter 7) in check.

Like other strains of *Bifidobacteria*, *B. breve* converts lactose and other sugars into nutrients and compounds your body can use. *B. breve* also helps break down plant fibers that normally would be indigestible.

B. lactis

One strain of *bifidobacteria, B. lactis,* is found in raw milk and is used as a starter culture for fermented milk products like buttermilk, cheese, and cottage cheese.

B. lactis is one of the most helpful good bacteria. Among other things, *B. lactis*

- Improves digestion.
- Enhances immune function.
- Can lower cholesterol.
- Promotes good oral health.
- Reduces inflammation and allergic responses.
- May help fight tumors.

B. longum

Researchers studying *Bifidobacterium longum* have discovered some very exciting properties of this strain of good bacteria. In addition to aiding in digestion, improving gut health, and boosting immunity, *B. longum* appears to help fight cancer. One study in rats with colon cancer found that *B. longum* prevented the tumors from growing and kept the cancer from spreading to other parts of the body.

B. longum also helps prevent antibiotic-related diarrhea (see Chapter 4) and eases symptoms of lactose intolerance. This good bacteria also may treat or prevent various kinds of allergies, high cholesterol, and inflammation associated with a number of digestive disorders.

Yogurt and other fermented dairy foods, as well as fermented vegetables like sauerkraut, are good food sources of *B. longum*.

Clostridium Difficile (Bad and Ugly)

Commonly known as *C. diff*, *Clostridium difficile* is a particularly nasty bacterium that seems to live everywhere — in the air, soil, and water, and in human and animal feces. *C. diff* spores can survive on surfaces for weeks or even months, and you can easily ingest them simply by touching a contaminated surface. A *C. diff* infection can cause diarrhea or even life-threatening inflammation in the colon.

C. diff seems to cause the most problems in hospitals and nursing homes, and it's a quite common side effect of taking antibiotics (see Chapter 4). The elderly and those with suppressed immune systems are most susceptible to *C. diff* infections. However, even otherwise healthy people can succumb.

Since 2000, a new strain of *C. diff* has arisen that is more resistant to certain drugs and produces more toxins than other strains. This stronger strain has shown up in patients who haven't been hospitalized or taken antibiotics. Careful hygiene — especially washing your hands thoroughly and frequently — is the best defense against all strains of *C. diff.*

Escherichia Coli (Bad)

Most *E. coli* strains are relatively harmless, and many of the harmful varieties cause nothing more than a brief bout of diarrhea. But some strains of this kind of bacteria can cause serious illness, including severe abdominal cramps, bloody diarrhea, and vomiting. Young children and older adults also are particularly susceptible to complications that can be life-threatening, such as kidney failure.

E. coli can contaminate food or water. Common sources of contamination include:

✔ **Fresh produce:** If water used to irrigate crops is contaminated with *E. coli*, the bacteria can in turn contaminate the produce. Although public water systems use chlorine to kill many harmful bacteria, private water supplies can be contaminated by human or animal waste runoff.

✔ **Ground beef:** When cattle are slaughtered for beef, bacteria from their intestines can contaminate the meat. Because ground beef uses meat from several individual cows, the risk of contamination is greater. Thoroughly cooking ground beef kills most harmful bacteria.

✔ **Raw milk:** *E. coli* can live on cows' udders and in milking equipment. Pasteurization kills the bacteria, but *E. coli* can be present in unpasteurized, or raw, milk.

Helicobacter Pylori (Bad)

H. pylori is associated with gastric ulcers and gastritis, and people who have *H. pylori* infections appear to have a slightly increased risk of developing stomach cancer — although the connection, if any, between stomach cancer and *H. pylori* isn't well understood.

The vast majority — 80 percent or more — of people who have *H. pylori* in their digestive systems have no symptoms, which leads some researchers to conclude that this potentially harmful bacteria is an important part of your gut flora. *H. pylori* infections are more common in developing countries than in industrialized nations.

Lactobacillus (Good)

Most lactic acid bacteria convert *lactose,* a sugar found in milk products, and other sugars into lactic acid, which your muscles use as fuel. In addition to being part of the gut flora, *Lactobacillus* also resides in the vagina and in the mouth.

Because *Lactobacillus* generates lactic acid, its environment is acidic, and that helps keep harmful bacteria at bay. In addition, *Lactobacillus* protects the lining of the vagina by building a barrier between pathogens and the lining, and it helps maintain the proper pH balance in the vagina (see Chapter 7 for more on good bacteria and women's health).

Some *Lactobacillus* strains may have therapeutic properties. Early research indicates some *Lactobacilli* (the plural form of *Lactobacillus)* can suppress inflammation and even prevent certain types of cancerous lesions in the colon and other organs.

For a century, scientists thought lactic acid build-up in the muscles was bad for you. The idea arose when Nobel laureate Otto Meyerhof put the bottom half of a frog in a jar and jolted the legs with electric shocks. After a few spasms, the muscles stopped moving, and when Meyerhof examined them, he saw that they were awash in lactic acid. His theory was that lack of oxygen to muscle tissue leads to a build-up of lactic acid, which in turn leads to muscle fatigue. Only recently have scientists learned that, in fact, muscles use lactic acid as fuel, and a build-up of lactic acid in muscle tissue means more energy for those muscles to work with.

L. Acidophilus (Good)

One of the Lactobacillus species, *L. acidophilus*, also lives in the intestine and vagina, helping with digestion and aiding in digestive health. In the vagina, *L. acidophilus* may help combat bacterial vaginosis (see Chapter 7), although clinical evidence isn't conclusive on that point yet.

L. acidophilus is commonly found in yogurt and fermented soy products, such as tempeh and miso.

Salmonella (Bad)

Salmonella is the most commonly reported bacterial infection, causing more than 1.4 million cases of food-borne illness and about 400 deaths every year in the United States. There are more than 2,300 strains of *Salmonella*; two strains, *Salmonella enteritidis* and *Salmonella Typhimurium,* are responsible for half of all human infections.

Salmonella passes through human or animal feces and can contaminate foods. Because this bacteria doesn't change the appearance, smell, or taste of food, it's easily ingested unknowingly.

Salmonella infections typically involve nausea and diarrhea. For mild cases, treatment typically consists of fluids to prevent dehydration. Sometimes doctors prescribe antidiarrheal medications and/or antibiotics, and severe cases can require hospitalization.

Shigella (Bad)

Shigella bacterial infections are most common in children between the ages of 2 and 4. Diarrhea, often bloody, is the main symptom of a *shigella* infection.

Like other diarrhea-causing bacteria, *shigella* can be contracted through direct contact with feces (as when changing diapers or helping toddlers with toilet training), so good hand-washing practices are important. *Shigella* also can be transmitted through contaminated food or by drinking or swimming in contaminated water.

Index

• H •

• I •

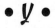
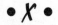

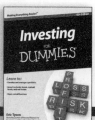
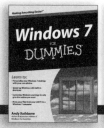
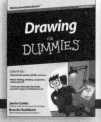
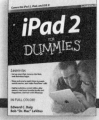

Math & Science

Algebra I
For Dummies,
2nd Edition
978-0-470-55964-2

Biology
For Dummies,
2nd Edition
978-0-470-59875-7

Chemistry
For Dummies,
2nd Edition
978-1-1180-0730-3

Geometry
For Dummies,
2nd Edition
978-0-470-08946-0

Pre-Algebra Essentials
For Dummies
978-0-470-61838-7

Microsoft Office

Excel 2010
For Dummies
978-0-470-48953-6

Office 2010 All-in-One
For Dummies
978-0-470-49748-7

Office 2011 for Mac
For Dummies
978-0-470-87869-9

Word 2010
For Dummies
978-0-470-48772-3

Music

Guitar
For Dummies,
2nd Edition
978-0-7645-9904-0

Clarinet For Dummies
978-0-470-58477-4

iPod & iTunes
For Dummies,
9th Edition
978-1-118-13060-5

Pets

Cats For Dummies,
2nd Edition
978-0-7645-5275-5

Dogs All-in One
For Dummies
978-0470-52978-2

Saltwater Aquariums
For Dummies
978-0-470-06805-2

Religion & Inspiration

The Bible
For Dummies
978-0-7645-5296-0

Catholicism
For Dummies,
2nd Edition
978-1-118-07778-8

Spirituality
For Dummies,
2nd Edition
978-0-470-19142-2

Self-Help & Relationships

Happiness
For Dummies
978-0-470-28171-0

Overcoming Anxiety
For Dummies,
2nd Edition
978-0-470-57441-6

Seniors

Crosswords
For Seniors
For Dummies
978-0-470-49157-7

iPad 2 For Seniors
For Dummies,
3rd Edition
978-1-118-17678-8

Laptops & Tablets
For Seniors
For Dummies,
2nd Edition
978-1-118-09596-6

Smartphones & Tablets

BlackBerry
For Dummies,
5th Edition
978-1-118-10035-6

Droid X2 For Dummies
978-1-118-14864-8

HTC ThunderBolt
For Dummies
978-1-118-07601-9

MOTOROLA XOOM
For Dummies
978-1-118-08835-7

Sports

Basketball
For Dummies,
3rd Edition
978-1-118-07374-2

Football
For Dummies,
2nd Edition
978-1-118-01261-1

Golf For Dummies,
4th Edition
978-0-470-88279-5

Test Prep

ACT For Dummies,
5th Edition
978-1-118-01259-8

ASVAB For Dummies,
3rd Edition
978-0-470-63760-9

The GRE Test
For Dummies,
7th Edition
978-0-470-00919-2

Police Officer Exam
For Dummies
978-0-470-88724-0

Series 7 Exam
For Dummies
978-0-470-09932-2

Web Development

HTML, CSS, & XHTML
For Dummies,
7th Edition
978-0-470-91659-9

Drupal For Dummies,
2nd Edition
978-1-118-08348-2

Windows 7

Windows 7
For Dummies
978-0-470-49743-2

Windows 7
For Dummies,
Book + DVD Bundle
978-0-470-52398-8

Windows 7 All-in-One
For Dummies
978-0-470-48763-1

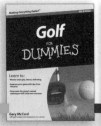
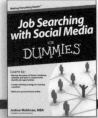
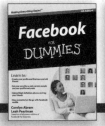
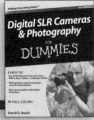

Available wherever books are sold. For more information or to order direct: U.S. customers visit
www.dummies.com or call 1-877-762-2974. U.K. customers visit www.wileyeurope.com or
call (0) 1243 843291. Canadian customers visit www.wiley.ca or call 1-800-567-4797.

Connect with us online at www.facebook.com/fordummies or @fordummies

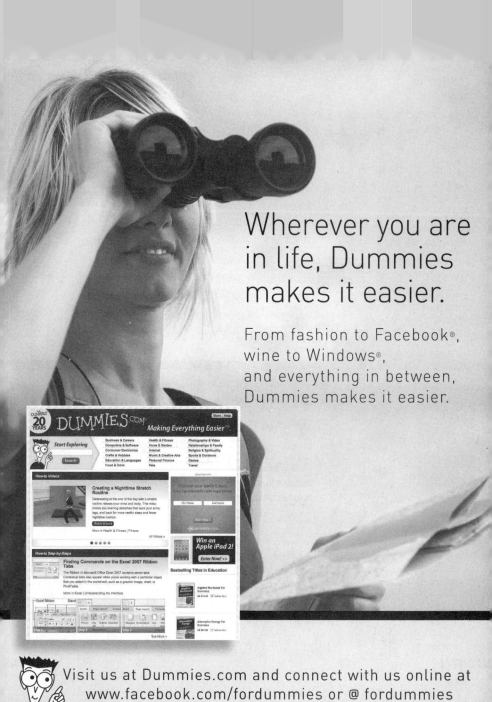

Wherever you are in life, Dummies makes it easier.

From fashion to Facebook®, wine to Windows®, and everything in between, Dummies makes it easier.

Visit us at Dummies.com and connect with us online at www.facebook.com/fordummies or @ fordummies

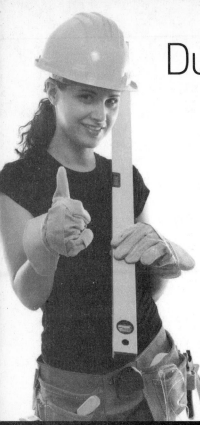
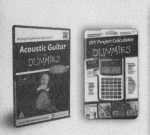
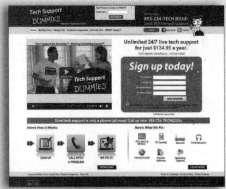
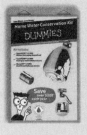
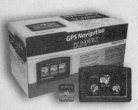
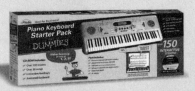
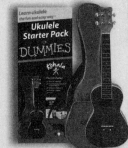
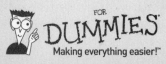

Why Choose Probulin?

1 Probulin is made with acid protection technology that minimizes the loss of bacteria due to harsh stomach acid.

2 Probulin is recommended by a prominent Gastroenterologist.

3 Probulin contains multiple bacteria, including Lactobacillus acidophilus DDS-1, one of the most researched strains of probiotics. In total, Probulin includes seven types of probiotic bacteria. More strains of bacteria are better than one. It is best if supplements include both Lactobacillus and Bifidobacter strains, as Probulin does.

4 Probulin uses the PREBIOTIC Inulin: a high-density plant-produced fiber. Prebiotics are food ingredients that help live bacteria grow and prosper. Probulin is the next generation in probiotics because it uses probiotics plus prebiotics to create a synbiotic.

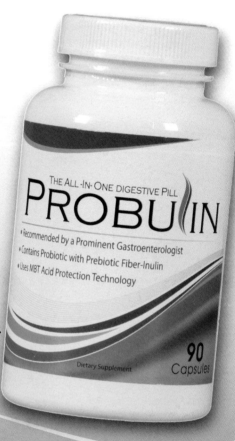

THE ALL-IN-ONE DIGESTIVE PILL
PROBULIN
• Recommended by a Prominent Gastroenterologist
• Contains Probiotic with Prebiotic Fiber-Inulin
• Uses MBT Acid Protection Technology

Dietary Supplement

90 Capsules

The next generation in probiotics

PROBULIN
"THE ALL-IN-ONE DIGESTIVE PILL"

FOR OPTIMAL DIGESTIVE HEALTH: Choose Probulin Today

www.Probulin.com | 1-855-PROBULIN (776-2854)

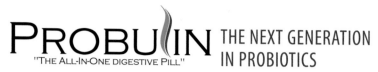

PROBU/IN
"THE ALL-IN-ONE DIGESTIVE PILL"

THE NEXT GENERATION IN PROBIOTICS

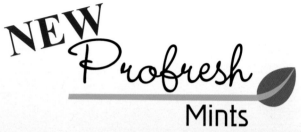

NEW *Profresh*
Mints

- Supports gum and tooth health
- Naturally freshens breath
- Gently whitens teeth

WWW.PROFRESHMINTS.COM

Natural Foods Containing Probiotics

YOGURT | Make sure it isn't pasteurized after fermentation, which kills the bacteria.

KEFIR | Made from cow, goat or sheep's milk, it is a sour drink fermented with kefir grains.

SAUERKRAUT | Cabbage fermented in brine, but must be raw to contain active cultures.

MISO | Fermented Japanese seasoning made from beans or grains.

PICKLES & OLIVES | Naturally contain probiotics only if not pasteurized.

TEMPEH | A source of vitamin B12, tempeh is a fermented grain made from soybeans.

KIMCHI | Another cabbage dish, it is a spicy & sour form of pickled sauerkraut.

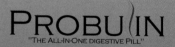

PROBU/IN
"THE ALL-IN-ONE DIGESTIVE PILL"

FOR OPTIMAL DIGESTIVE HEALTH: Choose Probulin Today

www.Probulin.com | 1-855-PROBULIN (776-2854)

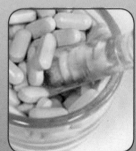

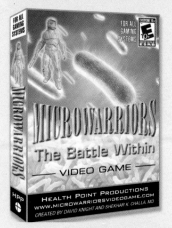
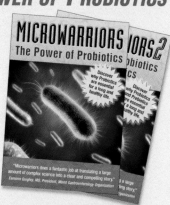
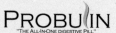